Fourth Edition

The Midwife's Pocket Formulary

T0195206

Fourth Edition

The Midwife's Pocket Formulary

Liz Davey PhD, BSc (Hons) Midwifery, PGDipEd, MA, RGN, RM, DPSM

Senior Lecturer in Midwifery,
Bournemouth University, Dorset, UK

Debbee Houghton BSc (Hons) Midwifery Practice, PGDipEd, MAHSCEd, RGN, RM, DPSN

Senior Lecturer in Midwifery,
Bournemouth University, Dorset, UK

ELSEVIER

Notices

ISBN: 978-0-7020-7861-3

Content Strategist: Alison Taylor/Poppy Garraway
Content Development Specialist: Kirsty Guest
Project Manager: Beula Christopher
Design: Ryan Cook

Printed in India

Last digit is the print number: 9   8   7   6   5   4   3   2

Working together
to grow libraries in
developing countries

www.elsevier.com • www.bookaid.org

Contents

Introduction

In contemporary midwifery practice, the midwife is required to provide a range of professional competencies and be proficient in clinical skills in order to promote safe childbirth for women. One of these proficiencies is medicines management, therefore midwives and students are required to have an understanding of the range of medicines used within their sphere of practice.

The Nursing and Midwifery Council have recently published the "Standards of proficiency for midwives" document (NMC 2019). Whilst all six domains reflect accountable and effective midwifery care, the shared skills for evidence based medicines administration and optimisation (principally Domains 3 and 4) essentially underpin all aspects of professional midwifery practice (NMC 2019 p40). These replace the "Standards for Medicines Management" (NMC 2007) which were withdrawn in January 2019.

The proficiency standards together with additional NMC and Royal Pharmaceutical Society publications (NMC 2015 and 2017; RPS 2018) aim to provide clear guidance and structure for the midwifery profession in all aspects of administration of medications, and directs the professional to use evidence to guide their monitoring and evaluation of medicines in the overall care plan. During undergraduate education, essential skills relating to medicines are integral to the curriculum ensuring competence at the point of professional registration.

The aim of this book is to provide a reference text and to guide routine and aspects of complex clinical practice.

The student should be aware of:

- the student's role in medicine management, medicines optimisation (National Institute for Health and Care Excellence (NICE) NG5 2015) and antimicrobial stewardship (Furber et al. 2017)

1

- medicines legislation
- the legal requirements of Midwives' Exemptions
- the differences and legal requirements between patient specific directions (PSDs) and patient group directions (PGDs)
- the midwives' supply order
- the drug schedules and legal requirements for medicines used in contemporary clinical practice, e.g. controlled drugs
- basic pharmacological principles – pharmacokinetics, pharmacodynamics, pharmacotherapeutics and pharmaceuticals (see Glossary).

Legal Classification of Medicines

The legal controls on the retail sale or supply of medicines are set out in the Medicines Act 1968 and The Human Medicines Regulations 2012 (and Amendments 2014 and 2016). Medicines are classified into three categories: Prescription-Only Medicine (POM), Pharmacy (P) or General Sales List (GSL). Each category is subject to a number of controls that apply to medicines sold or supplied by retail, or any other form of supply.

Prescription-Only Medicine (POM)

Section 58 of the Medicines Act 1968 Sections 214–219 of The Human Medicines Regulations 2012:

These medicines may be sold or supplied only from a registered pharmacy and in accordance with a prescription issued by an appropriate practitioner (a doctor, dentist, independent (nurse) prescriber, pharmacist independent prescriber or supplementary prescriber) (see Johnson and Taylor 2016).

Pharmacy (P)

Section 52 of the Medicines Act 1968 (see also Section 220 of The Human Medicines Regulations 2012):

Pharmacy medicines do not require a prescription and may be sold or supplied only in a registered pharmacy by or under the supervision/presence of a pharmacist. The package gives information on dosage (see Johnson and Taylor 2016).

General Sales List (GSL)

Section 53 of the Medicines Act 1968 (see also Sections 221–222 of The Human Medicines Regulation 2012):

These drugs are those that can be sold with reasonable safety without the supervision of a pharmacist, for example in a supermarket. However, they can be sold only from lockable premises and in the original manufacturers' packs (see Johnson and Taylor 2016).

Medicines unlicensed in the UK

Separate and additional national controls apply to the supply of a medicine that is not licensed for marketing within the UK. Such medicines cannot be advertised. A doctor can prescribe only where the patient has a special need that a licensed medicine cannot meet or where an appropriate licensed medicine is not available.

Midwives' Exemptions

Midwives at the point of registration can supply and/or administer, any of the substances that are specified in medicines legislation under the Midwives' Exemptions, provided this is in the course of their professional midwifery practice. "Midwives exemptions are distinct from prescribing, which requires the involvement of a pharmacist in the sale or supply of the medicine. Exemptions also differ from the arrangements for patient group directions (PGDs) as the latter must comply with specific legal criteria, be signed by a doctor or dentist and a pharmacist and authorised by an appropriate body" (NMC 2017, p. 18). If a medicine is not included in the Midwives' Exemptions then a prescription, PSD or a PGD is required (NMC 2017).

PGDs allow healthcare professionals to supply and administer specified medicines to pre-defined groups of patients, without a prescription (NICE 2013).

PSD is an instruction to administer a medicine to a list of individually named patients where each patient on the list has been individually assessed by that prescriber. The prescriber must have adequate knowledge of the patient's health, and be satisfied that the medicine to be administered serves the individual needs of each patient (Mulvenna 2016).

Administration of medicines on midwives; exemptions by student midwives

"All midwives who support, supervise and assess student midwives should ensure that they are familiar with the law in relation to the supply of medicines, including the list of midwives exemptions, in order to safely support and supervise student midwives who may administer medicines to women in their care. In respect to medicines legislation, student midwives can only administer medicines on the midwives' exemptions list, with the exclusion of controlled drugs, under the direct supervision of a midwife. Student midwives are not permitted to administer controlled drugs" (NMC 2017, p. 19) or PGDs (Human Medicines Regulations 2012).

References

Department of Health (DoH). (2010a). *Midwifery 2020: Delivering expectations*. London: DoH. Available from: https://www.gov.uk/govern ment/publications/midwifery-2020-delivering-expectations. [Accessed 12 April 2019].

Furber, C., Allison, D., & Hindley, C. (2017). *Antimicrobial resistance, antibiotic stewardship, and the role of the midwife's role. British Journal of Midwifery*, 25(11), 693–698.

Her Majesty's Stationary Office. (1968). *The medicines act 1968*. London: HMSO. Available from: https://www.legislation.gov.uk/ukpga/1968/67/ pdfs/ukpga_19680067_en.pdf. [Accessed 12 April 2019].

Her Majesty's Stationary Office. (1971). *The misuse of drugs act 1971*. London: HMSO. Available from: https://www.legislation.gov.uk/ukpga/ 1971/38/pdfs/ukpga_19710038_en.pdf. [Accessed 12 April 2019].

Her Majesty's Stationary Office. (2002). *The misuse of drugs regulations 2001*. London: HMSO. Available from: http://www.legislation.gov.uk/u ksi/2001/3998/pdfs/uksi_20013998_en.pdf. [Accessed 12 April 2019].

Her Majesty's Stationary Office. (2012). *The human medicines regulations 2012*. London: HMSO. Available from: http://www.legislation.gov.uk/uksi /2012/1916/pdfs/uksi_20121916_en.pdf. [Accessed 12 April 2019].

Her Majesty's Stationary Office. (2014). *The human medicines (amendment) regulations 2014*. London: HMSO. Available from: http://www.legislation.gov.uk/uksi/2014/490/pdfs/uksi_20140490_en.pdf. [Accessed 12 April 2019].

Her Majesty's Stationary Office. (2016). *The human medicines (amendment) regulations 2016*. London: HMSO. Available from: https://www.legislation.gov.uk/uksi/2016/186/pdfs/uksi_20160186_en.pdf. [Accessed 16 April 2019].

Johnson, R. & Taylor, W. (2016). *Skills for midwifery practice*. (4th ed.) Edinburgh: Elsevier.

Mulvenna, S. (2016). *Patient specific directions*. Available from: https://www.england.nhs.uk/south/wp-content/uploads/sites/6/2016/04/patient-specific-directions.pdf. [Accessed 5 July 2019].

National Health Service England (NHSE). (2015). *National maternity review: Better births. Improving outcomes of maternity services in England: a five year forward view for maternity care* [online]. London: NHSE. Available from: https://www.england.nhs.uk/wp-content/uploads/2016/02/national-maternity-review-report.pdf. [Accessed 5 July 2019].

National Institute for Health and Care Excellence (NICE). (2013). *MPG2 Patient group directions [online]*. Last updated March 2017 Available from: https://www.nice.org.uk/guidance/mpg2. [Accessed 5 July 2019].

National Institute for Health and Care Excellence (NICE). (2015). *NG5 Medicines optimisation: The safe and effective use of medicines to enable the best possible outcomes* [online]. Last updated March 2019. London, NICE. Available from: https://www.nice.org.uk/guidance/ng5 [Accessed 16 April 2019].

National Institute for Health and Care Excellence (NICE). (2016). *QS120 Medicines optimisation* [online]. London: NICE. Available from: https://www.nice.org.uk/guidance/qs120. [Accessed 16 April 2019].

Nursing and Midwifery Council (NMC). (2007). *Standards for medicines management*. Last updated April 2010. London: NMC. Available from: http://nipec.hscni.net/midwivesandmedicines/NMC-Standards-for-medicines-management.pdf. [Accessed 28 November 2019].

Nursing and Midwifery Council (NMC). (2015). *The Code - Professional standards of practice and behaviour for nurses, midwives and nursing associates*. update 2018. London: NMC.

Nursing and Midwifery Council (NMC). (2017). *Practicing as a midwife in the UK*. updated 2019. London: NMC.

Nursing and Midwifery Council (NMC). (2018). *Realising professionalism: Standards for education and training. Part 2: Standards for student supervision and assessment*. London: NMC.

Nursing and Midwifery Council (NMC). (2019). *Standards of proficiency for midwives*. London: NMC.

Royal Pharmaceutical Society (RPS). (2013). *Medicines optimisation: helping patients make the most of medicines*. Available from: https://www.rpharms.com/Portals/0/RPS%20document%20library/Open%20access/Policy/helping-patients-make-the-most-of-their-medicines.pdf. [Accessed 16 April 2019].

Royal Pharmaceutical Society (RPS). (2018). *Professional guidance on the safe and secure handling of medicines*. Available from: https://www.rpharms.com/recognition/setting-professional-standards/safe-and-secure-handling-of-medicines/professional-guidance-on-the-safe-and-secure-handling-of-medicines. [Accessed 12 April 2019].

Royal Pharmaceutical Society and Royal College of Nursing. (2019). *Professional guidance for the administration of medicines in healthcare settings*. London: Endorsed by RCM. RPS.

Abbreviations

b.d.	*bis die* – twice a day
t.d.s.	*ter die sumendus* – three times a day
q.d.s.	*quatre die sumendus* – four times a day
nocte	at night
stat	immediately
p.r.n.	*pro re nata* – as the need arises
IM	intramuscular – of injections
IV	intravenous
IVI	intravenous infusion
P.O.	per os – by mouth
P.R.	per rectum – rectally
P.V.	per vaginam – vaginally
S.C.	subcutaneous – of injections
mcg	microgram
mg	milligram
g	gram
kg	kilogram
mL	millilitre
L	litre
w/v	weight (of solute) per volume (of solvent)
ACE	Angiotensin converting enzyme
ADHD	Attention-deficit/hyperactivity disorder
ADR	Adverse drug reaction is an unwanted or harmful reaction which occurs after administration of a drug or drugs and is suspected or known to be due to the drug(s) (NICE Clinical Skills Summaries, 2017, Available from: https://cks.nice.org.uk/adverse-drug-reactions #!backgroundSub).
APTT	Activated partial prothrombin time – used to monitor clotting when anticoagulant used is heparin
ARM	Artificial rupture of membranes

AV	atrioventricular node
BNF	*British National Formulary* – information for healthcare professionals from an authoritative and practical focus that is regularly updated in published and online format. Available from: http://bnf.org/bnf/index.htm
BP	British Pharmaceutical
CD	Controlled drug
CHM	Commission on Human Medicines
CNS	Central nervous system
CPR	Cardiopulmonary resuscitation
DCT	Direct Coombes test
DVT	Deep vein thrombosis
ECG	electrocardiogram
eMC	*electronic Medicines Compendium* – information about UK-licensed medicines. Available from: http://www.medicines.org.uk/emc/
GABA	Gamma-aminobutyric acid – a deficiency of this inhibitory neurotransmitter may cause excessive responses to excitatory factors and may play a part in the initiation of abnormal discharge, and ultimately convulsions
GI	Gastrointestinal
GSL	General Sales List
GTN	Glyceryl trinitrate
HBIg	Hepatitis B immunoglobulin
HBsAg	Hepatitis B surface antigen
HDN	Haemorrhagic disease of the newborn
HIV	Human immunodeficiency virus
INR	International normalized ratio – usually used to monitor prothrombin time when anticoagulant used is warfarin
IUCD	Intrauterine contraceptive device
IUD	Intrauterine death

LAST	Local Anaesthetic Systemic Toxicity. Defined as any unusual cardiovascular or neurological signs or symptoms, including acute cardiac arrest, after administration of any local anaesthetic (LA) medication.
LMWH	Low molecular weight heparin
LSCS	Lower-segment caesarean section
MHRA	Medicines and Healthcare products Regulatory Agency
MAOI	Monoamine oxidase inhibitor – a drug that prevents the breakdown of serotonin, leading to an increase in mental and physical activity
MMR	Measles, mumps and rubella (vaccine)
MRP	Manual removal of placenta
MRSA	Methicillin-resistant *Staphylococcus aureus*
NB	nota bene (from the latin) or note well
NHS	National Health Service
NICE	National Institute of Health and Clinical Excellence
NSAID	Non-steroidal anti-inflammatory drug – a drug that inhibits the production of prostaglandins and that has antipyretic, anti-inflammatory and analgesic properties
OCP	Oral contraceptive pill
P	Pharmacy-only medicine
PCAS	Patient-controlled analgesia system
PDA	Patent ductus arteriosus
PE	Pulmonary embolus
PGD	Patient Group Direction is signed by a doctor and agreed by a pharmacist, which then acts as a direction to a nurse to supply and/or administer prescription-only medicines (POMs) to patients using their own assessment of patient need, without necessarily referring back to a doctor for an individual prescription.

PIL	Patient information leaflet, or PL – package leaflet
PND	Postnatal depression
PPH	Postpartum haemorrhage
PPHN	Persistent pulmonary hypertension in the newborn
POM	Prescription-only medicine
POP	Progestogen-only pill
PSD	Patient Specific Direction is the traditional written instruction, from a doctor, dentist, nurse, midwife or pharmacist, independent prescriber for medicines to be prescribed to a named patient
PT	Prothrombin time
RDS	Respiratory distress syndrome
RPS	Royal Pharmaceutical Society
SLE	Systemic lupus erythematosus
SPC or SmPC	Summary of product characteristics – reference document produced by pharmaceutical companies based on research and product knowledge to aid information to patients. These are approved by UK and European licensing agencies after checking product safety and efficacy
SRM	Spontaneous rupture of membranes
SSRI	Selective serotonin reuptake inhibitor – these drugs inhibit the reuptake of serotonin at nerve terminals, leading to inhibition of excitatory impulses and subsequent overload, and are used in conditions such as depression, anxiety and panic disorders
TCA	Tricyclic antidepressants – complex action but thought to inhibit the uptake and reuptake of serotonin and noradrenaline (norepinephrine)

UFH	Unfractionated heparin
URTI	Upper respiratory tract infection
UTI	Urinary tract infection
VZV	Varicella-zoster virus
WHO	World Health Organization

Glossary of Terms

Anticholinergic – a drug that inhibits the effects of acetylcholine, a chemical transmitter released by some nerve endings at the synapse between one neuron and another, or the nerve endings and effector organ. It supplies the lower motor neurons and parasympathetic nerves. Anticholinergic drugs relax smooth muscle, are antispasmodics, and inhibit secretory responses and vomiting.

Antimuscarinic – a synthetic anticholinergic drug; the opposite of a muscarinic drug.

Extrapyramidal – affecting the nerve tracts outside the pyramidal (spinal) tract.

Medication (Administration) Error or Incident (ME/MAE/MAI) – errors in medication administration which occur through failure in any of the 'five rights' (right patient, medication, time, dose, and route).

Mendelson syndrome – acid aspiration in obstetrical women during delivery, usually associated with general anaesthesia.

Muscarinic – causes sympathetic symptoms, i.e. the actions of acetylcholine on the nerve endings and the sympathetic nerves; for example, increases salivation, bronchial secretions, gastrointestinal activity.

Myasthenia gravis – an extreme form of muscle weakness, thought to be related to the rapid destruction of acetylcholine at neurotransmitter junctions.

Pharmaceutical drug – a medicine, medication, medicant or chemical substance used in diagnosis, treatment or prevention of disease.

Pharmacodynamics – actions of the medication on the body.

Pharmacokinetics – how the body handles the medication.

Pharmacotherapeutics – the effect of medication on the body.

Wernicke's encephalopathy – a neurological condition due to vitamin B_1 (thiamine) deficiency. In relation to midwifery care it may be seen in women with severe hyperemesis.

1

Anaesthesia

These drugs depress part of the central nervous system, causing the loss of sensation in a part of or in the whole of the body. There are two main groups, inhalational and intravenous.

These drugs are the specialty of an anaesthetist, although midwives do use certain ones, e.g. 50% nitrous oxide and 50% oxygen via Entonox™ apparatus (or piped supply), or local agents such as lidocaine for perineal infiltration and bupivacaine for epidural top-ups. This chapter explores the anaesthetics used by midwives and not those administered by anaesthetists alone. It is also of note that in the MBRRACE-UK (2018) Saving Lives, Improving Mother's Care 2014–2016 report, anaesthesia was given as the direct cause of death for one woman (0.04 per 100,000 maternities) (p6) reduced from two in the previous triennial review (2012–2014). Yet there is continued recommendation for improvement to overall care management by all professional groups (piv), especially where vulnerabilities and/or multiple health issues exist, and for women from Black and Asian ethnic backgrounds.

Midwives need to be aware of the action of anaesthetics, and maternity units need to provide recovery areas for women having a caesarean section and high-risk women.

The student should be aware of:

- the difference between analgesia and anaesthesia
- the difference between local, regional and general anaesthesia
- the physiology and pathophysiology of the perception of pain

- the physiological principles underpinning epidural anaesthesia
- problems that occur with obstetrical anaesthesia, i.e. the effects of progesterone on the mother, the presence of two patients rather than one, the pressure of the gravid uterus
- updated resuscitation techniques
- the key issues of LAST – see Chapter 15 and use of intralipid preparations in an emergency scenario
- how to apply cricoid pressure if requested to in an emergency.

BP
Nitrous oxide

Proprietary
Entonox™ (BOC Healthcare)

Group
Anaesthetic, inhalational

Uses/indications
Analgesia during labour

Type of drug
POM, Midwives' Exemptions or PGD

Presentation
Colourless gas with slightly sweet odour in cylinders – blue with blue and white quarters at the valve end and labelled Entonox. Cylinders should be: stored under cover; not stored near stocks of combustible materials. F size cylinders and larger should be stored vertically. D size cylinders are smaller, may be stored horizontally, but ensure cylinders are maintained at a temperature above 10°C for at least 24 hours before use to ensure the gases are mixed correctly. Care needed when handling and using gas-filled cylinders, including trans-portation – cylinders should be separate from the driver area, securely held, and emergency procedures known to the driver. Use of a hazard warning label is essential

---

Dosage

50% nitrous oxide : 50% oxygen, self-administered via mask or Entonox™ equipment

Route of admin

Inhalational

Contraindications

Pneumothorax, facial or jaw injuries, diving accidents, overt drunkenness

Side effects

Drowsiness and/or sedation, nausea, vomiting, middle ear damage or tympanic membrane damage (rare)

Interactions

None specific, but BNF [online] (2019) indicates that it may be appropriate to consider that nitrous oxide enhances the effect of other anaesthetics or analgesics, and is similar in action to a general anaesthetic. Relevant interactions to obstetrics are that:

Anxiolytics and hypnotics – enhances the sedative effect

Methyldopa – increases the hypotensive effect

Pharmacodynamic properties

Medical gas – colourless. Oxygen is an odourless gas and present in the atmosphere at 21%; nitrous oxide is a sweet smelling gas and potent analgesic from endorphin release when at 25% concentration, although a weak anaesthetic as the onset of effect and recovery are relatively rapid

Fetal risk

Can depress neonatal respiration (BNF [online] 2019). It is also of note that it may increase the risk of spontaneous abortion and low birthweight in female workers where levels of exposure are raised, i.e. operating theatres, labour wards

Breastfeeding

No data available on controlled studies during breastfeeding

BP
Lidocaine hydrochloride

Proprietary
Lidocaine hydrochloride 1% and 2% (Accord Health-care Ltd)
Lidocaine (non-proprietary, see BNF for details)

Group
Local anaesthetic

Uses/indications
Perineal infiltration – prior to episiotomy or suturing, **or for nerve blocks. Emergency use,** e.g. cardiac arrest – see Chapter 15 for indications, usage, and dosage

Type of drug
POM, Midwives' Exemptions or PGD

Presentation
Glass or polypropylene ampoules 2, 5, 10 or 20 mL, with strength 1% or 2%, indicated on the ampoule

Dosage
As per unit protocol, lowest concentration and smallest dose producing the required effect

Route of admin
Injection

Contraindications
Hypersensitivity, complete heart block and profound hypovolaemia

Side effects
Hypotension, bradycardia, hypersensitivity can lead to anaphylaxis, although this is rare; also inadvertent IV injection can lead to central nervous system excitatory response and then drowsiness, convulsions and respiratory arrest

Interactions

(Less likely when used topically.) **Anaesthetics** – action of suxamethonium is prolonged, bupivacaine increases the risk of myocardial depression. **Antacids** – cimetidine increases the plasma concentration absorption of lidocaine and can increase the risk of toxicity. **Antipsychotics** – increased risk of toxicity with myelosuppressive drugs. **β-blockers** – increased risk of myocardial depression with propranolol

Pharmacodynamic properties

Stabilizes the neuronal membrane and prevents the initiation and conduction of nerve impulses, causing profound anaesthesia of the membranes and lubrication that reduces friction. Effective in 5 min and lasts for 20–30 min

Fetal risk

Crosses placental barriers and can therefore cause after large doses neonatal respiratory depression, hypertonia, bradycardia after paracervical block, or accidental direct injection during infiltration of the perineum prior to episiotomy

Breastfeeding

Small amounts are secreted into breast milk, thus manufacturers indicate caution if used in nursing mothers

BP

Bupivacaine hydrochloride

Proprietary

Bupivacaine hydrochloride (anhydrous) 0.125% and 0.5% (ADVANZ Pharma)
Marcain Heavy® 0.5% w/v (Aspen)
Bupivacaine (non-proprietary, see BNF for details)

Group

Local anaesthetic

Uses/indications
Epidural anaesthesia, spinal anaesthesia

Type of drug
POM

Presentation
Polypropylene ampoules (Steripacks) of differing percentages

Dosage
As prescribed by the anaesthetist

Route of admin
Intrathecal injection

Contraindications
Hypovolaemia, hypotension, pyrexia in labour, pyogenic infection of the skin at or adjacent to the lumbar site, coagulation disorders or ongoing coagulation treatment, known hypersensitivity to local anaesthetics such as lidocaine, meningitis, hypovolaemic shock, intracranial haemorrhage, ventricle arrhythmias, cardiogenic shock, low levels of platelets

Side effects
Anaphylaxis, maternal hypotension, bradycardia – preloading with crystalloids required – persistent or profound symptoms can be reversed with ephedrine 10–15 mg IV (eMC 24/9/2019), myocardial depression and seizures if given IV, may cause maternal pyrexia and some diminishing of uterine contractions, post-lumbar headache. A high block causes respiratory embarrassment, arrest and paralysis, neurological problems include paraesthesia, motor weakness and loss of sphincter control; accidental IV injection – causes numbness of the tongue, tinnitus, light-headedness, dizziness and tremors, followed by drowsiness, convulsions and cardiac disorders, and requires the attendance of skilled anaesthetic help (LAST – see Chapter 15 and the use of intralipid preparations in an emergency scenario)

Interactions
Antiarrhythmics – increased myocardial depression

Pharmacodynamic properties
Marcain Heavy® – local anaesthetic of the amide type that causes moderate relaxation of lower extremities and a motor blockade of abdominal muscles.
Bupivacaine hydrochloride – properties as above, but analgesia without the motor blockade

Fetal risk
Reportedly bradycardia, respiratory depression, fetal hypothermia; toxicity in animal studies indicates avoidance in early pregnancy, but manufacturers suggest there is no evidence of untoward effects

Breastfeeding
Excreted in small amounts but no risk from therapeutic doses

BP
Lidocaine hydrochloride 2.5% and Prilocaine 2.5%

Proprietary
Emla™ 5% Cream (Aspen)

Group
Anaesthetic – local

Uses/indications
Anaesthesia prior to venepuncture, surface analgesia

Type of drug
POM

Presentation
White soft cream

Dosage
Thick layer 1–5 hours prior to procedure under occlusive dressing

Continued

Route of admin
Topical

Contraindications
Dermatitis at site, mucous membrane, wounds or hypersensitivity to active constituents

Side effects
Transient paleness, redness and oedema have been reported

Interactions
As for lidocaine, but unlikely

Pharmacodynamic properties
Provides dermal analgesia, depending on application time and dose, by causing transient local vasoconstriction or vasodilation at the treated area

Fetal risk
Crosses the placental barrier, but no ill effects have been reported

Breastfeeding
Excreted in breast milk in small amounts but considered safe

BP
Lidocaine hydrochloride 2% and Chlorhexidine gluconate 0.25%

Proprietary
Instillagel® (CliniMed)

Group
Anaesthetic – local (surface anaesthesia)

Uses/indications
Anaesthesia of the urethra prior to catheterization, or topical application to mucous membranes, i.e. the perineum

Type of drug
POM

Presentation
Ampoules of gel or in accordion gel pack

Dosage
6 or 11 mL intraurethrally to fill urethra

Route of admin
Topical/intraurethral

Contraindications
Hypersensitivity to lidocaine. Trauma to the urethra can cause increased systemic absorption

Side effects
As for lidocaine but fewer, as topically applied

Interactions
As for lidocaine, but unlikely

Pharmacodynamic properties
Stabilizes the neuronal membrane and prevents the initiation and conduction of nerve impulses, causing profound anaesthesia of the membranes and lubrication that reduces friction. Effective in 5 min and lasts for 20–30 min

Fetal risk
No evidence of harm but avoid in early pregnancy

Breastfeeding
No evidence of risk

References and Recommended Reading

Briggs, G., Freeman, R., Towers, C., & Forinash, A. (2017). *Drugs in pregnancy and lactation: A reference guide to fetal and neonatal risk* (11th ed.). Philadelphia: Wolters Kluwer.

British Oxygen Corporation [BOC was British Oxygen Company which combined with Linde to form The Linde Group in 2006]. (2015). *Entonox. BOC Medical Gas Datasheet (MGDS)*. Available from: https://www.bochealthcare.co.uk/en/images/HLC_505605-MGDS%20ENTONOX%20%28web%29_tcm409-57640.pdf. [Accessed 19 April 2019].

Howie, L., & Rankin, J. (2017). Pain relief in labour. In J. Rankin (Ed.), *Physiology in childbearing with anatomy and related biosciences* (4th ed.) (pp. 399–410). Edinburgh: Elsevier.

Instillagel gel. *Clinimed Ltd.* Last updated on the BNF [online] April 2019.

Jackson, K., Marshall, J., & Brydon, S. (2014). Physiology and care during the first stage of labour. In J. Marshall, & M. Raynor (Eds.), *Myles textbook for midwives* (16th ed.) (pp. 349–356). Edinburgh: Churchill Livingstone/Elsevier. 327–366. See specifically the section: Woman's control of pain during labour.

Jordan, S. (2010). Pain relief. In S. Jordan (Ed.), *Pharmacology for midwives: The evidence base for safe practice* (2nd ed.). Basingstoke: Palgrave Macmillan.

MBRRACE-UK. (2018). *MBRRACE-UK: Saving lives, improving mothers' care. Lessons learned to inform maternity care from the UK and Ireland. Confidential enquiries into maternal deaths and morbidity 2014–16.* Oxford: MBRRACE/NPEU. Available from https://www.npeu.ox.ac.uk/mbrrace-uk/reports. [Accessed 12 April 2019].

Nursing and Midwifery Council (NMC). (2019). *Standards of proficiency for midwives*. London: NMC. Available from: https://www.nmc.org.uk/globalassets/sitedocuments/standards/standards-of-proficiency-for-midwives.pdf. [Accessed 20 November 2019].

Rang, H., Ritter, J., Flower, R., & Henderson, G. (2016). *Rang and Dale's pharmacology* (8th ed.). Edinburgh: Elsevier Churchill Livingstone.

SmPC from the eMC. Bupivacaine hydrochloride 0.125% and 0.5% solution for injection. ADVANZ Pharma. Last updated on the eMC 24/4/2019.

SmPC from the eMC. Emla™ cream 5%. Aspen. Last updated on the eMC 4/5/2017.

SmPC from the eMC. Lidocaine 1% and 2% solution for injection. Accord Healthcare Ltd. Last updated on the eMC 11/12/2017.

SmPC from the eMC. Marcain Heavy 0.5% w/v solution for injection. Aspen. Last updated on the eMC 16/3/2018.

Tsen, L. (2010). Neuroxial analgesia and anaesthesia in pregnancy. In D. James, P. Steer, C. Weiner, B. Gonik, & S. Robson (Eds.), *High risk pregnancy: Management options* (5th ed.) (pp. 1811–1842). Cambridge: Cambridge University Press.

Vamer, R. G. (1993). Mechanisms of regurgitation and its prevention with cricoid pressure. *International Journal of Obstetrical Anaesthesia, 2*, 207–215.

Weiner, C., & Mason, C. (2017). Medication. In D. James, P. Steer, C. Weiner, B. Gonik, & S. Robson (Eds.), *High risk pregnancy: Management options* (5th ed.) (pp. 808–846). Cambridge: Cambridge University Press.

Further Reading

Armstrong, S., & Fernando, R. (2013). Analgesics and anti-inflammatory, general and local anaesthetics and muscle relaxants. In D. Mattison (Ed.), *Clinical pharmacology during pregnancy* (pp. 129–144). Edinburgh: Elsevier.

Berlin, C. (2013). Medications and the breastfeeding mother. In D. Mattison (Ed.), *Clinical pharmacology during pregnancy* (pp. 41–54). Edinburgh: Elsevier.

Boyle, M., & Bothamley, J. (2018). *Critical care assessment by midwives.* London: Routledge.

Herbert, M. (2013). Impact of pregnancy on maternal pharmacokinetics of medications. In D. Mattison (Ed.), *Clinical pharmacology during pregnancy* (pp. 17–40). Edinburgh: Elsevier.

National Institute of Health and Care Excellence (NICE). (2019). *NG121 Intrapartum care for women with existing medical conditions or obstetric complications and their babies [online].* London: NICE. Available from https://www.nice.org.uk/guidance/ng121. [Accessed 14 April 2019].

National Institute of Health and Care Excellence (NICE). (2014). *CG190 Intrapartum care for healthy women and babies [online].* London: NICE. Last updated February 2017. Available from https://www.nice.org.uk/guidance/cg190. [Accessed 14 April 2019].

2

Analgesics

These preparations are used to relieve pain without causing unconsciousness or lack of all nervous sensation in a particular area. It is important to become familiar with pain theories and to use the body's natural analgesics to their optimum effect, as well as using chemical preparations.

The student should be aware of:

■ pain theories, especially the 'gate theory' of Melzack and Wall (1964) and recent theories on the 'neuromatrix' understanding of pain
■ the difference between anaesthesia and analgesia
■ the accumulative effect of many analgesics, which can lead to intentional or accidental overdose
■ the different combinations of separate analgesic compounds
■ the possibility of addiction to analgesics
■ the evidence-based guidance on the use of codeine for antenatal and postnatal analgesia in light of MHRA guidance (RCOG 2018)
■ neonatal sequelae to maternal analgesia
■ the appropriateness of the analgesic compound to the complaint.

BP
Paracetamol (Acetaminophen)

Proprietary
Paracetamol (Zentiva and Typharm Ltd) (refer to BNF
for manufacturers and advice on trade names)
Calpol® infant suspension (McNeil Products Ltd;
Pinewood Healthcare) (refer to BNF for manufacturers
and advice on trade names)

Group
Analgesic, non-opioid

Uses/indications
Mild to moderate pain, including headache, rheumatic
pain, pyrexia, dysmenorrhea, toothache, sore throat
and colds

Type of drug
POM, GSL (sold to the public in packs of no more than
16 tablets; pharmacists may dispense up to 32 tablets;
also sold as infant suspension or sugar-free infant
suspension, as 100 mL or 200 mL bottles or packets of
12 × 5 mL sachets), often authorized by PGD

Presentation
Tablets, oral suspension, dispersible tablets, suppositories

Dosage
Adult: Oral: 500 mg–1 g 4–6 hourly (max 4 g daily)
(eMC 3/8/2018); P.R.: 0.5–1 g q.d.s. (eMC 5/9/2017)
Paediatric: Oral – dose calculated on 10 mg per kg
body weight (eMC 4/4/2019)

Route of admin
Oral, P.R.

Contraindications
Hypersensitivity, hepatic and renal disease, alcohol
dependence

Continued

Side effects
Rare, blood disorders, rashes, overdose causes liver damage recorded at levels of 10 mg but at 5 mg in some cases, pancreatitis with prolonged use

Interactions
Anticoagulants – with prolonged use seems to enhance effect of warfarin. *Cholestyramine* – reduces the absorption of paracetamol. *Metaclopromide* – enhances the effect of paracetamol.

Pharmacodynamic properties
Antipyretic, peripherally acting analgesic

Fetal risk
Epidemiological studies in human pregnancy show no ill effects

Breastfeeding
Short courses only – amount secreted too small to be harmful. No controlled study data available and taken by a large number of women with no observed increase in adverse effects on breastfed infants, therefore considered safe

---

BP
Aspirin (Acetylsalicylic acid)

Proprietary
Aspirin (Accord-UK Ltd)
Resprin Suppositories (Martindale Pharma)
(Various generic manufacturers; see BNF for advice)

Group
Analgesic, non-opioid, NSAID

Uses/indications
Mild to moderate pain, including headache, neuralgia, rheumatic pain, transient musculoskeletal pain, pyrexia

Type of drug
GSL (sold to the public in packs of no more than 16 tablets; pharmacists may dispense up to 32 capsules/tablets), POM

Presentation
Tablets, some dispersible, suppositories

Dosage
Oral: 300–600 mg 3–4 hourly, max 12 tablets or 3.6 g per day (eMC 8/7/2013)

P.R: 2–3 suppositories every 4 hours (eMC 7/11/2018). Not more than 12 suppositories to be used in any 24 hours

Route of admin
Oral, P.R.

Contraindications
Hypersensitivity, clotting disorders, haemophilia, asthma, angio-oedema, urticaria, rhinitis, impaired renal or hepatic function, dehydration, gastric ulceration, pregnancy, unless in very low doses on obstetrician's orders

Side effects
Increased bleeding time, leading to potential haemorrhage, i.e. antepartum, intrapartum, postpartum, delayed onset and duration of labour (low doses are not harmful), mild and infrequent gastric irritation/ulceration, hypersensitivity, bronchospasm and skin reactions in hypersensitive patients, haematuria, nervousness, dizziness, tinnitus, insomnia, rash

Continued

Interactions

Alcohol – enhanced effect on the gut. *Antacids* – increased alkalinity of urine. *Analgesics* – concomitant admin increases side effects. *Anticoagulants* – increased risk of haemorrhage (potentiates antiplatelet effect). *Antiepileptics* – enhanced effect of phenytoin and valproate. *Corticosteroids* – enhances the risk of gastrointestinal bleeding and ulceration. *Metoclopramide* – increases rate of absorption and therefore increased effects of aspirin.

Pharmacodynamic properties

Aspirin is an analgesic, antipyretic, anti-inflammatory that inhibits the synthesis of prostaglandins

Fetal risk

Low-dose aspirin is not thought to have harmful effects; in high doses: closure of PDA in utero, persistent pulmonary hypertension, possible reduction in the amount of amniotic fluid (Weiner and Mason, 2017) not recommended after 34 weeks' gestation, kernicterus in jaundiced neonates; is also reported to be linked with fetal growth deficiency and a purpuric rash in neonates, with depression of the platelet function

Breastfeeding

Low quantities of salicylates and of their metabolites are excreted into the breast milk – not thought to be significant for short-term use, regular high doses could cause impairment of platelet function and hypoprothrombinaemia if neonatal vitamin K stores are low. Acetylsalicylic acid may be a contributory factor in the causation of Reye's syndrome in some under 16 years old.

BP
Codeine phosphate

Proprietary
Codeine phosphate (Wockhardt UK Ltd)
Codeine phosphate injection (Torbay and North
Devon Healthcare Trust as Torbay Pharmaceuticals)
Codeine phosphate (non-proprietary, see BNF for details)

Group
Analgesic, opioid – morphine salt

Uses/indications
Mild to moderate pain, cough suppressant – NB:
Codeine should be used at the lowest effective dose
for the shortest period of time

Type of drug
POM (CD – injection)

Presentation
Tablets, syrup, ampoules (CD)

Dosage
Oral: 30–60 mg 4 hourly (max 240 mg daily)
(eMC 18/4/2017)
IM: 30–60 mg 4 hourly (eMC 14/7/2017)

Route of admin
Oral, IM

Contraindications
As for morphine, raised intracranial pressure

Side effects
Constipation, nausea, sedation, respiratory depression, especially cough reflex, dependence. In labour –
maternal gastric stasis and increased risk of inhalation
pneumonia

Interactions
As for diamorphine

Continued

Pharmacodynamic properties
Codeine is a narcotic analgesic that acts via the central nervous system

Fetal risk
First trimester: inguinal hernias, cardiac, circulatory and respiratory system defects, cleft lip and palate, although not according to Weiner and Mason (2017); second trimester: alimentary tract defects; labour: neonatal respiratory depression and withdrawal

Breastfeeding
Not recommended (see RCOG review clarification of pain relief options 2018). Codeine should not be used during breastfeeding. Codeine exerts its effect through μ opioid receptors, although codeine has low affinity for these receptors, and its analgesic effect is due to its conversion to morphine.

BP
Co-codaprin

Proprietary
Co-codaprin dispersible tablets (Accord-UK Ltd)
Co-codaprin (non-proprietary, see BNF for details)

Group
Analgesic, aspirin compound (aspirin 400 mg + codeine phosphate 8 mg)

Uses/indications
Mild to moderate pain

Type of drug
POM

Presentation
Tablets (white)

Dosage
1–2 tablets 4–6 hourly (max 8 daily) (emC 13/11/2018)

Route of admin
Oral

Contraindications
As for codeine and aspirin

Side effects
As for codeine and aspirin

Interactions
As for codeine and aspirin

Fetal risk
As for codeine and aspirin

Breastfeeding
Not recommended (see RCOG review clarification of pain relief options 2018). Codeine should not be used during breastfeeding.

BP
Co-dydramol (Paracetamol 500 mg + Dihydrocodeine 10 mg)

Proprietary
Co-dydramol tablets 10/500 mg (Wockhardt UK Ltd)
co-dydramol (non-proprietary, see BNF for details)

Group
Analgesic, paracetamol and opioid (dihydrocodeine) compound

Uses/indications
Mild to moderate pain

Type of drug
POM, GSL

Presentation
Tablets (white)

Continued

Dosage
1–2 tablets 4–6 hourly, max 8 per day (eMC 25/5/2017)

Route of admin
Oral

Contraindications
As for paracetamol and dihydrocodeine

Side effects
As for paracetamol and dihydrocodeine

Interactions
As for paracetamol and dihydrocodeine

Fetal risk
As for dihydrocodeine

Breastfeeding
Not recommended (see RCOG review clarification of pain relief options 2018). Codeine should not be used during breastfeeding.
Distalgesic

BP
Co-codamol (Paracetamol 500 mg + Codeine Phosphate 8 mg or Paracetamol 500 mg + Codeine Phosphate 30 mg)

Proprietary
Co-codamol 8/500 and 30/500 tablets (Zentiva) – paracetamol 500 mg + codeine phosphate hemihydrate 8 mg or 30 mg
Co-codamol (non-proprietary, see BNF for details)

Group
Analgesic, paracetamol and opioid compound

Uses/indications
Mild to moderate pain

Type of drug
POM, P

Presentation
Tablets, capsules, dispersible tablets

Dosage
1–2 tablets or capsules 4 hourly, max 8 per day
(eMC 5/9/2018)

Route of admin
Oral

Contraindications
As for paracetamol and codeine

Side effects
As for paracetamol and codeine phosphate

Interactions
As for paracetamol and codeine phosphate

Fetal risk
As for codeine phosphate

Breastfeeding
Not recommended (see RCOG review clarification of
pain relief options 2018). Codeine should not be used
during breastfeeding.

BP
Ibuprofen

Proprietary
Brufen® (Mylan Ltd) (GSL – Nurofen®, Crookes
Healthcare Ltd)
Ibuprofen (non-proprietary, see BNF for details)

Group
Analgesic, non-opioid, NSAID

Uses/indications
Mild to moderate pain, particularly perineal

Type of drug
POM, (GSL)

Presentation
Tablets, syrup, granules

Dosage
1.2–1.8 g daily in 3–4 doses (after food) (eMC
14/12/2018)

Route of admin
Oral

Contraindications
Pregnancy, salicylate hypersensitivity, asthma

Side effects
Gastrointestinal discomfort, diarrhoea, nausea, rash,
headache, dizziness

Interactions
As for diclofenac and salicylic acid

Pharmacodynamic properties
Analgesic, anti-inflammatory, antipyretic; this NSAID is
thought to act by inhibiting prostaglandin synthesis

Fetal risk
As for salicylic acid, delayed onset and increased duration of labour

Breastfeeding
Limited studies suggest NSAIDs can appear in the
breast milk in very low concentrations; manufacturer
recommends avoid during breastfeeding

BP
Mefenamic acid

Proprietary
Ponstan™ (Chemidex Pharma Ltd)
Mefenamic acid (non-proprietary, see BNF for details)

Group
Analgesic, non-opioid, NSAID

Uses/indications
Mild to moderate pain, postpartum pain, postoperative pain, anti-inflammatory

Type of drug
POM

Presentation
Tablets, capsules

Dosage
500 mg t.d.s. after food (eMC 3/1/2016)

Route of admin
Oral

Contraindications
Hypersensitivity to mefenamic acid, irritable bowel syndrome, peptic/intestinal ulceration, renal or hepatic impairment, asthma or allergic reactions, i.e. rhinitis or urticaria or bronchospasm on administration of NSAIDs

Side effects
Drowsiness, diarrhoea, nausea, rash, thrombocytopenia, haemolytic anaemia or purpuric rash. If these occur withdraw the drug; hypersensitive reaction – bronchospasm, urticaria, nausea, vomiting, abdominal pain, headache, facial oedema, laryngeal oedema, dizziness, abnormal vision, palpitations

Interactions
As for diclofenac, but especially:
Anticoagulants – increased effect
Antihypertensives – reduces the hypotensive effect
OVERDOSE – can cause convulsions

Continued

Pharmacodynamic properties
A prostaglandin synthesis inhibiting NSAID with anti-inflammatory, antipyretic effects and analgesic properties

Fetal risk
Safety is not established and possibly has same effects as salicylic acid; known effects of NSAIDs on the fetal cardiovascular system (risk of closure of the ductus arteriosus); use in the last trimester of pregnancy is contraindicated

Breastfeeding
Trace amounts may be present in breast milk and transmitted to the infant; therefore manufacturers recommend against use during breastfeeding

---

BP
Diclofenac sodium

Proprietary
Diclofenac sodium tablets (Dexcel Pharma Ltd)
Dicloflex (Dexcel Pharma Ltd)
Voltarol® suppositories (Novartis Pharmaceuticals UK Ltd)
Diclofenac sodium (non-proprietary, see BNF for details)

Group
Analgesic, non-opioid, NSAID

Uses/indications
Moderate to severe pain, musculoskeletal pain, used post LSCS, anti-inflammatory properties

Type of drug
POM, Midwives' Exemptions

Presentation
Tablets some dispersible, ampoules, suppositories

Dosage

Oral: 75–150 mg daily in divided doses, preferably after food (max 150 mg in 24 hours) (eMC 3/1/2018)
P.R.: 100 mg 18–24 hourly (max 150 mg in 24 hours) (eMC 7/4/2017)
Rarely – deep IM: 75 mg daily (max 2 days) (see BNF 2019)

Route of admin

Oral, P.R., rarely deep IM

Contraindications

Asthma, pregnancy, hypersensitivity to NSAIDs, may exacerbate crohn's disease or ulcerative colitis, cardiac, hepatic or renal impairment, clotting disorders, e.g. pph

Side effects

Uterine inertia, delayed onset and increased duration of labour, increased postpartum blood loss, coagulation disorders leading to haemorrhage, asthma, bronchospasm, gastric irritability/ulceration, rectal irritation, headache, dizziness, vertigo, abdominal pain, rash, purpura, urticaria, drowsiness, disturbances of vision, loss of sensation, malaise, fatigue and insomnia

Interactions

Analgesics – concomitant admin, causes increased side effects. *Antihypertensives* – calcium channel blockers; antagonizes hypotensive effects. *β-blockers* – antagonism of hypotensive effects. *Methlydopa* – antagonism of the hypotensive effect. *Anticoagulants – coumarins* – anticoagulant effect is increased. *Heparin* – increased risk of haemorrhage with IV diclofenac *Antiepileptics* – phenytoin – possible enhanced effect. *Zidovudlne* increased risk of haematological toxicity

Pharmacodynamic properties

NSAID analgesic that inhibits prostaglandin synthesis, with antipyretic properties

Continued

Fetal risk

Benefits must outweigh the risk and the lowest possible effective dose should be used; can cause closure of PDA in utero, persistent pulmonary hypertension

Breastfeeding

Amount secreted too small to be harmful and evidence of risk is remote, although there are only a limited number of controlled studies in breastfeeding women

---

BP

Diamorphine hydrochloride

Proprietary

Diamorphine Hydrochloride Injection (Wockhardt UK Ltd)
Diamorphine hydrochloride (non-proprietary, see BNF for details)

Group

Analgesic – morphine salt – narcotic acting primarily on the central nervous system and smooth muscle

Uses/indications

Moderate to severe pain, i.e. postoperative and labour

Type of drug

POM, CD authorized by PGD and Midwives' Exemptions

Presentation

Tablets, powder for reconstitution or pre-diluted ampules

Dosage

5–10 mg 4 hourly (depending on woman's size)
(eMC 14/12/2015)
Slow IV injection: 0.25–0.5 of the corresponding IM dose (eMC 14/12/2015)

Route of admin

IM, oral, slow IV injection

Contraindications

Existing respiratory depression, asthma, raised intracranial pressure as it affects papillary responses, phaeochromocytoma – endogenous release of histamines may stimulate catecholamine release

Side effects

Gastric stasis in labour, sedation, nausea, vomiting, respiratory depression, dependence, tachycardia, hypothermia, hallucinations, mood swings, facial flushing, sweating, constipation, dizziness, miosis, confusion, urinary retention, biliary spasm, postural hypotension, vertigo, palpitations, dry mouth, urticaria, pruritus, raised intracranial pressure and rarely circulatory depression

Interactions

Non-specific to diamorphine but characteristic of opioids. *Alcohol* – enhances the sedative effect, increases hypotension. *Analgesics* – enhanced effects. *Antidepressants* – avoid concurrent administration of MAOI or administration within 2 weeks of their discontinuation increases the sedative effect of tricyclics. *Anxiolytics and hypnotics* – enhances the sedative effect. *Cimetidine* – inhibits metabolism, thereby increasing the plasma concentration of the opioid. *Metoclopramide* – antagonism of the effect on gastrointestinal activity

Pharmacodynamic properties

Narcotic analgesic acting on the central nervous system (CNS) and smooth muscle. Its predominant action is to depress the CNS, but it has stimulant actions resulting in nausea, vomiting and miosis

Fetal risk

Crosses the placental barrier within 1 hour of administration; causes withdrawal symptoms, respiratory depression, meconium aspiration, intrauterine death

Breastfeeding
Therapeutic doses are unlikely to affect the infant, but in dependent mothers secretion into breast milk may cause problems with withdrawal and addiction

BP
Morphine sulfate

Proprietary
Oramorph® (Boehringer Ingelheim Ltd)
Morphine sulfate (Wockhardt UK Ltd)
Morphine sulfate (non-proprietary, see BNF for details)

Group
Analgesic – narcotic

Uses/indications
Postoperative pain, to potentiate epidural anaesthesia, patient-controlled analgesia systems (PCAS)

Type of drug
POM, P, CD authorized by PGD and Midwives' Exemptions

Presentation
Oral solution, tablets, capsules, suspension, suppositories, ampoules

Dosage
IM or S.C.: 10–15 mg 4 hourly (depending on patient size, severity of pain, response and tolerance to dosage) (eMC 10/1/2019)
Slow IV injection: 0.25–0.5 of IM dose (eMC 10/1/2019)
Intrathecal: dosage determined by anaesthetist
PCAS: determined by hospital protocols; post LSCS usage is increasing, refer to BNF but typically 10–20 mL 3 hourly
P.R.: 15–30 mg 4 hourly (see BNF 2019)
Oral: recommended dose 10-20 mg (5-10 mL) every 4 hours, max 120 mg per day (see BNF 2019)

Route of admin
Oral, IM, S.C., P.R., IV, intrathecal

Contraindications
Renal or hepatic impairment, respiratory depression, asthma, raised intracranial pressure (affects papillary responses), phaeochromocytoma

Side effects
As for diamorphine. NB: postoperative patients should be observed closely for delayed or rebound respiratory depression as well as other side effects

Interactions
As for diamorphine

Pharmacodynamic properties
Morphine is a narcotic analgesic obtained from opium; acts on the central nervous system and smooth muscle

Fetal risk
As for diamorphine and pethidine

Breastfeeding
Therapeutic doses unlikely to affect the infant and so considered moderately safe

---

BP
Fentanyl

Proprietary
Fentanyl citrate (hameln pharmaceuticals ltd)
Fentanyl citrate (non-proprietary, see BNF for details)

Group
Analgesic, opioid – morphine salt

Uses/indications
Enhancement of anaesthesia, i.e. epidural

Type of drug
CD

Presentation
Pre-diluted ampoules, premixed solution in polybags of 100 or 200 mL for intrathecal infusion in continuous epidurals

Dosage
50–200 mcg individualised to patient weight, age and condition, subsequent doses 50 mcg p.r.n. (eMC 15/4/2019)

Route of admin
Intrathecal (IM or IV not used in obstetrics)

Contraindications
Caution in existing respiratory depression, myasthenia gravis, known hypersensitivity to fentanyl or opioids

Side effects
Respiratory depression – can be delayed, apnoea, transient hypotension, bradycardia, nausea, vomiting, itching, muscular rigidity, myoclonic movements, urinary retention. Hypersensitivity can cause anaphylaxis

Interactions
As for morphine

Pharmacodynamic properties
A synthetic opiate with 50–100 times the clinical potency of morphine; has a rapid onset but duration of action is short. Its peak effect is at 30 min post dosage; differs from morphine in its short duration of action and its lack of emetic effect

Fetal risk
No evidence of teratogenic or embryotoxic effects, but manufacturers advise avoidance. Crosses the placental barrier and may cause loss of fetal heart variability without fetal hypoxia, respiratory depression or withdrawal symptoms, although these may be less via intrathecal route

Breastfeeding
No controlled study data available. Although it is likely to be present in trace amounts in breast milk and breastfeeding is not recommended for 24 hours after administration, there is no evidence of an increased risk of adverse effects in breastfed infants

---

BP
Dihydrocodeine tartrate

Proprietary
Dihydrocodeine (Accord-UK Ltd)
Dihydrocodeine injection (Martindale Pharma, an Ethypharm Group Company)
Dihydrocodeine (non-proprietary, see BNF for details)

Group
Analgesic, opioid – morphine salt

Uses/indications
Moderate to severe pain

Type of drug
POM (CD – injection)

Presentation
Tablets (white), elixir, ampoules (CD)

Dosage
Oral: 30 mg 4–6 hourly (preferably after food), higher doses cause nausea and vomiting (eMC 8/7/2019)
Deep S.C., IM: 50 mg repeated 4–6 hourly
(eMC 26/9/2014)

Route of admin
Oral, IM, deep S.C.

Contraindications
Raised intracranial pressure, respiratory difficulties

Continued

Side effects
Constipation, drowsiness, respiratory depression, hypotension, dizziness, dependence; high doses cause nausea and vomiting

Interactions
As for diamorphine

Pharmacodynamic properties
Dihydrocodeine is a semi-synthetic narcotic analgesic with a potency between that of morphine and codeine; acts on the opioid receptors in the brain to reduce the patient's perception of pain and improve the psychological reaction to pain by removing associated anxiety

Fetal risk
Little evidence to suggest fetal risk; however, there may be withdrawal symptoms, or respiratory depression in the neonate, and manufacturer advises use only when the benefits outweigh the risks

Breastfeeding
It is likely that dihydrocodeine is excreted in breast milk; therefore manufacturers advise avoidance

---

BP
Pethidine hydrochloride

Proprietary
Pethidine Hydrochloride (Martindale Pharma, an Ethypharm Group Company)
Pethidine hydrochloride (non-proprietary, see BNF for details)

Group
Analgesic – opioid, alkaloid

Uses/indications
Moderate to severe pain, obstetric analgesia

Type of drug
POM, CD authorized by PGD and Midwives' Exemptions

Presentation
Tablets, ampoules

Dosage
S.C./IM: 25–100 mg individualised to patient weight, age and condition, 4 hourly (eMC 10/7/2019)
Oral: 50–150 mg 4 hourly
Slow IV injection: 25–50 mg 4 hourly

Route of admin
IM, S.C., slow IV injection. Oral – rarely in obstetrics

Contraindications
Existing respiratory depression, renal impairment, pre-existing morphine addiction, compromised fetus

Side effects
Nausea, vomiting, respiratory depression, convulsions after overdose, bradycardia, dependence

Interactions
As for diamorphine. **Antacids** – cimetidine inhibits metabolism of pethidine

Pharmacodynamic properties
Pethidine binds to opioid receptors and exerts its principal pharmacological actions on the central nervous system where its analgesic and sedative effects are of particular therapeutic value. The respiratory depression produced by pethidine can be antagonized by naloxone and nalorphine. Similar to diamorphine

Fetal risk
Crosses placental barrier within 2 min of administration and present in amniotic fluid in 30 min; bradycardia, respiratory depression, withdrawal symptoms, slow excretion by neonatal liver

Breastfeeding
Depresses suck reflex, as for diamorphine

BP
Meptazinol hydrochloride

Proprietary
Meptid Injection (Almirall Ltd)

Group
Analgesic – opioid of hexahydroazepine group – narcotic

Uses/indications
Moderate to severe pain, i.e. postoperative, renal colic and labour

Type of drug
POM, CD authorized by PGD

Presentation
Solution for injection

Dosage
IM (eMC 24/9/2018) 75–150 mg 2–4 hourly (calculated from 2 mg/kg)
Slow IV injection 50–100 mg 2–4 hourly as required (eMC 24/9/2018)

Route of admin
IM, slow IV injection

Contraindications
Existing respiratory depression, asthma, raised intracranial pressure as it affects papillary responses, phaeochromocytoma – endogenous release of histamines may stimulate catecholamine release, MAOI medication and for 14 days post discontinuation – CNS excitation/depression with hypertension/hypotension, acute alcoholism

Side effects

Gastric stasis in labour, sedation, nausea, vomiting, respiratory depression, dependence, tachycardia, hypothermia, hallucinations, mood swings, facial flushing, sweating, constipation, dizziness, miosis, confusion, urinary retention, biliary spasm, postural hypotension, vertigo, palpitations, dry mouth, urticaria, pruritus, raised intracranial pressure and rarely circulatory depression

Interactions

Non-specific to diamorphine but characteristic of opioids, **Alcohol** – enhances the sedative effect, increases hypotension. **Analgesics** – enhanced effects. **Antidepressants** – avoid concurrent administration of MAOI; administration within 2 weeks of their discontinuation increases the sedative effect of tricyclics. **Anxiolytics and hypnotics** – enhances the sedative effect. **Cimetidine** – inhibits metabolism, thereby increasing plasma concentration of the opioid. **Metoclopramide** – antagonism of the effect on gastrointestinal activity

Pharmacodynamic properties

Centrally acting analgesic of the hexahydroazepine group acting on the CNS and smooth muscle. Predominant action is on opioid receptors, specifically those that have affinity to endogenous opioids (μ δ κ); effects only partly reversed by naloxone

Fetal risk

Crosses the placental barrier within 1 hour of administration; respiratory depression, meconium aspiration, intrauterine death

Breastfeeding

Therapeutic doses are unlikely to affect the infant, but manufacturers recommend that benefit should outweigh the risks

BP
Hyoscine butylbromide

Proprietary
Buscopan® tablets (SANOFI)
Hyoscine injection
Hyoscine (non-proprietary, see BNF for details)

Group
Antimuscarinics

Uses/indications
Gastrointestinal smooth muscle spasm, irritable bowel, diverticular disease, dysmenorrhoea

Type of drug
POM, P (GSL – sold to the public provided a single dose does not exceed 20 mg and the daily dose 80 mg; packs are restricted to 240 mg max)

Presentation
Tablets, ampoules

Dosage
Oral: 20 mg q.d.s. (eMC 11/10/2019)
IM, IV injection: 20 mg repeated after 30 min if required (eMC 15/10/2019)

Route of admin
Oral, IM, IV injection

Contraindications
Myasthenia gravis, paralytic ileus

Side effects
Constipation, transient bradycardia followed by tachycardia, palpitations, arrhythmias, urinary urgency and retention, photophobia, dry mouth, flushing and skin dryness; rarely – nausea, vomiting, giddiness, confusion

Interactions

Alcohol – enhances sedative effect of hyoscine.
Antidepressants – tricyclics have increased side effects
Antihistamines – increase the antimuscarinic side effects.
MAOIs – increased antimuscarinic effects
Phenothiazines – chlorpromazine increases the anti-muscarinic side effects

Pharmacodynamic properties

Antispasmodic agent that relaxes the smooth muscle of the organs of the abdominal and pelvic cavities, and acts on the intramural parasympathetic ganglia of these organs

Fetal risk

Animal studies show teratogenicity, but there are no controlled studies in pregnant women. Not recommended by manufacturer unless benefits outweigh the risks

Breastfeeding

Not recommended by manufacturer, but considered moderately safe as there are no observed increases in adverse effects in breastfed infants

BP

Remifentanil hydrochloride

Proprietary

Ultiva for Injection (Aspen)
Remifentanil powder for concentrate solution for injection/infusion (Hospira UK Ltd)
Remifentanil (non-proprietary, see BNF for details)

Group

POM

Uses/indications

Analgesia and sedation

Type of drug
Analgesic agent for use during induction and/or maintenance of general anesthesia by suitably qualified anesthetist in fully equipped setting for ventilation and cardiovascular support

Presentation
Lyophilised powder for reconstitution for IV administration

Dosage
Induction of anesthetic usually 1 mcg/kg body weight over at least 30 seconds; continuous infusion 0.5–1 mcg/kg/min (eMC 18/12/2018 and 15/4/2019)

Route of admin
Bolus injection or continuous infusion

Contraindications
Known hypersensitivity to remifentanil and other fentanyl analogues

Side effects
Opiate dependency, hypotension and bradycardia, respiratory depression, apnoea, muscle rigidity

Interactions
Beta-blockers and **calcium channel blocking agents** likely to exacerbate hypotension and bradycardia

Pharmacodynamic properties
Remifentanil is a selective μ-opioid agonist with a rapid onset and very short duration of action. The μ-opioid activity of remifentanil is antagonized by narcotic antagonists, such as naloxone.

Fetal risk
Remifentanil crosses the placental barrier and fentanyl analogues can cause respiratory depression in the fetus/neonate

Breastfeeding
Not known whether remifentanil is excreted in human milk

References and Recommended Reading

Armstrong, S., & Fernando, R. (2013). Analgesics and anti-inflammatory, general and local anaesthetics and muscle relaxants. In D. Mattison (Ed.), *Clinical pharmacology during pregnancy* (pp. 129–144). Edinburgh: Elsevier.

Bisson, D., Newell, S., & Laxton, C. (2018). *Scientific impact paper 59: Antenatal and postnatal analgesia*. [online]. London: RCOG. Available from: https://obgyn.onlinelibrary.wiley.com/doi/full/10.1111/1471-0528.15510. [Accessed 16 May 2019].

Briggs, G., Freeman, R., Towers, C., & Forinash, A. (2017). *Drugs in Pregnancy and Lactation: A reference guide to fetal and neonatal risk* (11th ed.). Philadelphia: Wolters Kluwer.

Griffiths, R. (2010). Law, medicines and the midwife. In S. Jordan (Ed.), *Pharmacology for midwives: The evidence base for safe practice* (2nd ed.) (pp. 62–74). Basingstoke: Palgrave Macmillan.

Johnson, R., & Taylor, W. (2016). *Skills for Midwifery Practice* (4th ed.). Edinburgh: Elsevier.

Jordan, S. (2010). Pain relief. In S. Jordan (Ed.), *Pharmacology for midwives: The evidence base for safe practice* (2nd ed.) (pp. 77–130). Basingstoke: Palgrave Macmillan.

National Institute for Health and Care Excellence (NICE). (2015). NG5 Medicines optimisation: the safe and effective use of medicines to enable the best possible outcomes [online]. Last updated March 2019. London: NICE. Available from: https://www.nice.org.uk/guidance/ng5 [Accessed 16 April 2019].

National Institute for Health and Care Excellence (NICE). (2016). QS120 *Medicines optimisation* [online]. Available from: https://www.nice.org.uk/guidance/qs120 [Accessed 16 April 2019].

Nursing and Midwifery Council (NMC), 2019. *Standards of proficiency for midwives*. London: NMC. Available from: https://www.nmc.org.uk/globalassets/sitedocuments/standards/standards-of-proficiency-for-midwives.pdf [Accessed 20 November 2019].

Rang, H., Ritter, J., Flower, R., & Henderson, G. (2016). *Rang and Dale's pharmacology* (8th ed.). Edinburgh: Elsevier Churchill Livingstone.

SmPC from the eMC. Aspirin 300mg tablets. Accord UK Ltd. Last updated on the eMC 8/7/2013.

SmPC from the eMC. Brufen® 400mg tablets. Mylan Ltd. Last updated on the eMC 14/12/2018.

SmPC from the eMC. Buscopan® 10 mg tablets as hyoscine butylbromide. SANOFI. Last updated on the eMC 11/10/2019.

SmPC from the eMC. Buscopan® 20 mg/mL injection. SANOFI. Last updated on the eMC 15/10/2019.

SmPC from the eMC. Calpol® infant suspension and infant suspension sachets. McNeil Products Ltd. Last updated on the eMC 4/4/2019.

SmPC from the eMC. Co-codamol 8mg/500mg tablets and Co-codamol 30mg/500mg tablets. Zentiva. Last updated on the eMC 5/9/2018.

SmPC from the eMC. Codeine Phosphate 30mg tablets. Wockhardt UK Ltd. Last updated on the eMC 18/4/2017.

SmPC from the eMC. Codeine Phosphate 60mg in 1mL solution for injection. Torbay and North Devon Health Care Trust as Torbay Pharmaceuticals. Last updated on the eMC 14/7/2017.

SmPC from the eMC. Co-dydramol 10mg/500mg tablets. Wockhardt UK Ltd. Last updated on the eMC 25/5/2017.

SmPC from the eMC. Diamorphine Hydrochloride 10mg for injection. Wockhardt UK Ltd. Last updated on the eMC 14/12/2015.

SmPC from the eMC. Diclofenac Sodium 50mg gastro-resistant tablets. Dexcel Pharma Ltd. Last updated on the eMC 2/1/2018.

SmPC from the eMC. Dicloflex 75mg tablets. Dexcel Pharma Ltd. Last updated on the eMC 3/1/2018.

SmPC from the eMC. Dihydrocodeine 30mg tablets. Accord-UK Ltd. Last updated on the eMC 8/7/2019.

SmPC from the eMC. Dihydrocodeine 50mg/mL injection. Martindale Pharma, an Ethypharm Group Company. Last updated on the eMC 26/9/2014.

SmPC from the eMC. Dispersible Co-codaprin tablets BP 8/400mg. Accord-UK Ltd. Last updated on the eMC 13/11/2018.

SmPC from the eMC. Fentanyl 50mcg/mL injection. hameln pharmaceuticals Ltd. Last updated on the eMC 15/4/2019.

SmPC from the eMC. Meptid 100mg as meptazinol hydrochloride injection. Almirall Ltd. Last updated on the eMC 24/9/2018.

SmPC from the eMC. Morphine Sulfate 10mg/mL injection. Wockhardt UK Ltd. Last updated on the eMC 10/1/2019.

SmPC from the eMC. Nurofen 200 mg tablets. Rickett Benckiser Healthcare (UK) Ltd. Last updated on the eMC11/7/2018.

SmPC from the eMC. Oramorph 10mg/5mL oral solution. Boehringer Ingelheim Ltd. Last updated on the eMC 8/4/2019.

SmPC from the eMC. Pethidine hydrochloride 50mg/mL and 100mg/2mL injection. Martindale Pharma, an Ethypharm Group Company. Last updated on the eMC 10/7/2019.

SmPC from the eMC. Ponstan forte 500mg tablets. Chemdex Pharma Ltd. Last updated on the eMC 3/1/2016.

SmPC from the eMC. Paracetamol 500mg capulets, tablets and soluble tablets. Zentiva. Last updated on the eMC 3/8/2018.

SmPC from the eMC. Paracetamol 500mg suppositories. Typharm Ltd. Last updated on the eMC 5/9/2017.

SmPC from the eMC. Remifentanil 2mg powder for concentrate for injection/infusion. Hospira UK Ltd. Last updated on the eMC 26/10/2018.

SmPC from the eMC. Resprin 300mg suppositories. Martindale Pharma. Last updated on the eMC 7/11/2018.

SmPC from the eMC. Ultiva 2mg for injection/infusion. Aspen. Last updated on the eMC 18/12/2018.

SmPC from the eMC. Voltarol® 12.5mg, 25mg, 50mg and 100mg suppositories. Novartis Pharmaceuticals UK Ltd. Last updated on the eMC 7/4/2017.

Weiner, C. & Mason, C., (2017). Medication. In D. James, P. Steer, C. Weiner, B. Gonik & S. Robson, (Eds.), *High risk pregnancy: Management options*. (5th ed.). Cambridge: Cambridge University Press. 808–846.

Further Reading

Wee, M., Tuckey, J., Thomas, P., & Burnard, S. (2013). A comparison of intramuscular diamorphine and intramuscular pethidine for labour analgesia: a two-centre randomized blinded controlled trial. *British Journal of Obstetrics and Gynaecology (BJOG)*, 121, 447–456.

Weibel, S., Jelting, Y., Afshari, A., Pace, N., Eberhart, L., Jokinen, J., et al. (2017). Patient-controlled analgesia with remifentanil versus alternative parenteral methods for pain management in labour. *Cochrane Database of Systematic Reviews* (Issue 4), CD011989. Available from: https://www.cochranelibrary.com/cdsr/doi/10.1002/14651858.CD011989.pub2/epdf/full. [Accessed 16 May 2019].

Wilson, M., MacArthur, C., Hewitt, C., Handley, K., Gao, F., Beeson, L., et al. (2018). Intravenous remifentanil patient-controlled analgesia versus intramuscular pethidine for pain relief in labour (RESPITE): an open-label, multicentre, randomised controlled trial. *The Lancet*, 392(10148), 662–672. Available from: www.thelancet.com/journals/lancet/article/PIIS0140-6736(18)31613-1/fulltext. [Accessed 16 May 2019].

3

Antacids

These drugs/preparations are used to reduce gastric acidity and give relief from heartburn when changes in diet and posture have no effect. They may also be used as prophylaxis prior to the induction of anaesthesia where there is a risk of Mendelson syndrome, i.e. before either elective or emergency caesarean section.

Antacids should not be taken at the same time as other medication as they impair absorption.

H_2 antagonists act on histamine receptors and can intensify or aggravate an asthmatic response. They should be used with caution in hepatic and or renal impairment.

The student should be aware of:

- the effect of progesterone on the mother
- local protocols for management of high-risk clients during labour
- the procedure of applying 'cricoid pressure' during induction of anaesthesia
- updated resuscitation techniques
- the effects of narcotic analgesia on gastric emptying.

BP
Cimetidine

Proprietary
Tagamet (Chemidex Pharma Ltd)
Cimetidine (non-proprietary, see BNF for details)

Group
Antacid, H_2 receptor antagonist

Uses/indications
To reduce gastric acidity, intrapartum or prior to caesarean section

Type of drug
POM

Presentation
Tablets – light green, also chewable and effervescent, syrup

Dosage
Oral – 400 mg at start of labour repeated 4 hourly (max 2.4 g/day) (eMC 7/11/2018)

Route of admin
Oral

Contraindications
Hypersensitivity to cimetidine, avoid in clients stabilized on phenytoin and warfarin

Side effects
Rare but include dizziness, rash, in high doses reversible confusional states, headache

Interactions
Analgesics – inhibits the metabolism of opioid analgesics and increases their plasma concentration
Antibiotics – inhibits the metabolism of metronidazole and erythromycin
Anticoagulants – inhibits the metabolism of warfarin, and enhances its effects
Antiepileptics – inhibits the metabolism of phenytoin, sodium valproate and carbamazepine
Antihypertensives – inhibits the metabolism of labetalol

Continued

Pharmacodynamic properties
H_2 receptor antagonist that rapidly inhibits both basal and stimulated gastric secretion of acid. It also reduces pepsin output

Fetal risk
No evidence to suggest cimetidine is hazardous, but it should be avoided unless necessary

Breastfeeding
Excreted in breast milk but not known to be harmful

BP
Ranitidine

Proprietary
Ranitidine tablets (Accord Healthcare Ltd)
Zantac injection (GlaxoSmithKlein UK)
Ranitidine (non-proprietary, see BNF for details)

Group
Antacid, H_2 antagonist

Uses/indications
Reduces gastric acidity in high-risk labours, prior to caesarean section or any other surgical procedure. Prophylaxis of acid aspiration (Mendelson) syndrome: 150 mg oral dose can be given 2 hours before anaesthesia, and preferably also 150 mg the previous evening. Alternatively, the injection is also available. In obstetric patients in labour, 150 mg every 6 hours, but if general anaesthesia is required it is recommended that a non-particulate antacid, e.g. sodium citrate, be given in addition. The usual precautions to avoid acid aspiration should also be taken.

Type of drug
POM, often authorized by PGD

Presentation
Tablets (also dispersible or effervescent), syrup, injection

Dosage
150 mg at onset of labour, repeat 6 hourly or see protocols (eMC 2/5/2017)
IM or slow IV 50 mg 45–60 min prior to the induction of analgesia (eMC 26/10/2015)

Route of admin
Oral, IM, IV injection

Contraindications
As for cimetidine, hypersensitivity

Side effects
As for cimetidine, rarely tachycardia, and with long-term use agitation and visual disturbances

Interactions
As for cimetidine, but effects less likely

Pharmacodynamic properties
As for cimetidine, relatively long-acting. Ranitidine is a specific, rapidly acting, histamine H_2 antagonist. It inhibits basal and stimulated secretion of gastric acid, reducing both the volume and the acid and pepsin content of the secretion. Ranitidine has a relatively long duration of action and so a single 150 mg dose effectively suppresses gastric acid secretion for 12 hours.

Fetal risk
Crosses the placenta and should only be used in the long term if essential, for prophylaxis in labour or LSCS. No adverse effect has been reported on labour, delivery or neonatal period

Breastfeeding
Excreted in breast milk, manufacturers recommend only if essential

BP
Alginic acid

Proprietary
Gaviscon Advance (Forum Health Products Ltd) –
aniseed or peppermint flavor
Alginic acid (non-proprietary, see BNF for details)

Group
Antacid – alginate

Uses/indications
Dyspepsia, cardiac reflux (heartburn)

Type of drug
GSL

Presentation
Tablets, oral suspension – aniseed or peppermint

Dosage
Tablets 1–2 as required, or 5–10 mL as required
(eMC 17/10/2014)

Route of admin
Oral

Contraindications
Hypersensitivity

Side effects
No data available, but caution in a sodium-restricted diet

Interactions
Impaired absorption of oral iron

Pharmacodynamic properties
Alginic acid reacts with the gastric acid to form a
pH-neutral gel raft over the stomach contents and is
effective for up to 4 hours

Fetal risk
Nil known from research studies, although manufacturer recommends limit treatment as much as possible

Breastfeeding
Not secreted in breast milk

References and Recommended Reading

Berlin, C. (2013). Medications and the breastfeeding mother. In D. Mattison (Ed.), *Clinical pharmacology during pregnancy* (pp. 41–54). Edinburgh: Elsevier.

Briggs, G., Freeman, R., Towers, C., & Forinash, A. (2017). *Drugs in pregnancy and lactation: A reference guide to fetal and neonatal risk* (11th ed.). Philadelphia: Wolters Kluwer.

Herbert, M. (2013). Impact of pregnancy on maternal pharmacokinetics of medications. In D D. Mattison (Ed.), *Clinical pharmacology during pregnancy* (pp. 17–40). Edinburgh: Elsevier.

Jordan, S. (2010). Management of gastric acidity in pregnancy. In S. Jordan (Ed.), *Pharmacology for midwives: The evidence base for safe practice* (2nd ed.) (pp. 263–270). Basingstoke: Palgrave Macmillan.

Jordan, S., & MacDonald, S. (2017). Pharmacology and the midwife. In S. MacDonald, & G. Johnson (Eds.), *Mayes' midwifery: A text book for midwives* (15th ed.) (pp. 158–174). Edinburgh: Elsevier.

National Institute of Health and Care Excellence (NICE). (2011). *CG132. Caesarean section [online]. Last updated August 2012. London: NICE.* https://www.nice.org.uk/guidance/cg132. [Accessed 14 April 2019].

Nursing and Midwifery Council (NMC), 2019. *Standards of proficiency for midwives. London: NMC. Available from:* https://www.nmc.org.uk/globalassets/sitedocuments/standards/standards-of-proficiency-for-midwives.pdf [Accessed 20 November 2019].

SmPC from the eMC. Cimetidine 200mg/5mL oral solution. Rosemont Pharmaceuticals Limited. Last updated on the eMC 14 June 2013.

SmPC from the eMC. Gaviscon Advance® – aniseed or peppermint. Forum Health Products Limited. Last updated on the eMC 17 October 2014.

SmPC from the eMC. Ranitidine® 150mg film-coated tablets. Accord Healthcare Ltd Last updated on the eMC 2 May 2017.

SmPC from the eMC. Tagamet® 200mg tablets. Chemidex Pharma Ltd. Last updated on the eMC 7 November 2018.

SmPC from the eMC. Zantac® 50mg/2mL injection. GlaxoSmithKline UK. Last updated on the eMC 26 October 2015.

Weiner, C., & Mason, C. (2017). Medication. In D. James, P. Steer, C. Weiner, B. Gonik, & S. Robson (Eds.), *High risk pregnancy: Management options* (5th ed.) (pp. 808–846). Cambridge: Cambridge University Press.

Vamer, R. G. (1993). Mechanisms of regurgitation and its prevention with cricoid pressure. *International Journal of Obstetrical Anaesthesia*, *2*, 207–215.

Further Reading

MBRRACE–UK. (2018). MBRRACE-UK: *Saving Lives, Improving Mothers' Care. Lessons learned to inform maternity care from the UK and Ireland. Confidential Enquiries into Maternal Deaths and Morbidity 2014–16.* Oxford: MBRRACE/NPEU. https://www.npeu.ox.ac.uk/mbrr ace-uk/reports. [Accessed 12 April 2019].

Paranjothy, S., Griffiths, J., Broughton, H., Gyte, G., Brown, H., & Thomas, J. (2014). Interventions at caesarean section for reducing the risk of aspiration pneumonitis. *Cochrane Review, Issue 2.* Art. No.: CD004943 https://www.cochranelibrary.com/cdsr/doi/10.1002/14651858.CD0049 43.pub4/full. [Accessed 22 May 2019].

4

Antibiotics

Antimicrobial agents stop the growth of microbes or kill microorganisms. Four specific representative groups are: antibiotics which act on bacteria, antifungals (Chapter 9) which are used against fungal infections, antivirals (Chapter 19) for treating viral infections and antiseptic chemicals (Chapter 12) for skin/mucous membrane application.

Antibiotics may be naturally produced by certain bacteria or fungi that interfere with or prevent the growth of other bacteria/ fungi. Others may be industrially produced by fermentation, semi-synthetic or synthetic techniques. They are used in the treatment of infection or as prophylaxis, e.g. in cases of spontaneous rupture of membranes longer than 24 hours, Group B Strep during labour, significant pyrexia in labour or lower-segment caesarean section.

The student should be aware of:

- causes and transmission of infection
- causal organisms of infection and their laboratory identification
- the symptoms and progression of infection including the increased risk of candidiasis colonisation
- the importance of bacterial culture and sensitivity
- the ingestion, uptake, action and excretion of the prescribed drug
- the NICE guideline on prophylaxis for infective endocarditis (CG 64) (2008 updated 2016), which recommended that antibiotics should not be given for dental or other interventional procedures, e.g. obstetrical/gynaecological procedure(s) or childbirth
- the guidance for common infections (NICE/PHE 2019) and specific group B streptococcal, chorioamnionitis, and endometritis guidance in maternity settings

- preterm pre-labour rupture of membranes guidance
- the diagnosis, management and treatment guidance for maternal sepsis in childbearing (RCOG CG64a and CG64b 2012; MBRRACE-UK 2018)
- the importance of antimicrobial stewardship in maternity care (NICE 2015) and the difference between antibiotic and antimicrobial resistance

---

BP
Metronidazole

Proprietary
Flagyl® (SANOFI)
Metronidazole infusion (Baxter Healthcare Ltd)
Metronidazole (non-proprietary, see BNF for details)

Group
Antimicrobial

Uses/indications
Treatment of anaerobic infection with a wide range of activity, prophylaxis in surgery (anaerobic bacteria and anaerobic streptococci), clostridium, *Trichomonas vaginalis, Eubacterium, Gardnerella vaginalis,* puerperal sepsis, bacterial vaginosis, gingivitis

Type of drug
POM

Presentation
Tablets, suspension, suppositories, pre-prepared IV injections and infusions

Dosage
Oral: stat 800 mg then 400–500 mg t.d.s. (eMC 23/10/2018)
IV infusion: 500 mg t.d.s. (eMc 11/2/2018)
P.R.: 1 g t.d.s. for 3 days max, then 1 g b.d. treatment of bacterial vaginosis as for oral, or 2 g single dose (eMC 23/10/2018)

Route of admin
Oral, P.R., IV, IM

Contraindications
In pregnancy and breastfeeding avoid high dosage, avoid alcohol, known hypersensitivity to metronidazole

Side effects
Unpleasant taste in mouth, furry tongue, nausea, vomiting, rashes, headache, drowsiness, dizziness, dark urine and, very rarely, angio-oedema

Interactions
Alcohol – disulfiram-like reaction – avoid during treatment and for 48 hours post course
Antacids – cimetidine inhibits the metabolism of metronidazole
Anticoagulants – enhances the effect of warfarin but no interaction with heparin
Antiepileptics – inhibits the metabolism of phenytoin; phenobarbital accelerates metabolism of metronidazole
Oestrogens – reduces the effect of the combined oral contraceptive pill

Pharmacodynamic properties
Antimicrobial effective against a wide range of infections with antiprotozoal and antibacterial actions

Fetal risk
Avoid high-dose regimens; use in first trimester can cause midline facial defects, cardiac defects, genital defects and limb defects, but has been used with little effect in last two trimesters

Breastfeeding
Significant amounts secreted; avoid large single doses

BP
Erythromycin stearate

Proprietary
Erythrocin® (ADVANZ Pharma)
Eythromycin lactobionate for injection (ADVANZ Pharma)
Erythromycin (non-proprietary, see BNF for details)

Group
Antibiotic, macrolide

Uses/indications
Used in penicillin-sensitive clients, penicillin-resistant organisms, syphilis, chlamydia, gonorrhoea, respiratory infection, treatment of infection sensitive to erythromycin, prophylaxis in management of pre-term rupture of membranes

Type of drug
POM

Presentation
Tablets, capsules, powder for reconstitution, granules, suspension

Dosage
1–2 g/day in even doses, depending on the severity of infection
Oral: 250–500 mg q.d.s. or 0.5–1 g b.d. (eMC 14/2/2018)
Syphilis/chlamydia: 500 mg q.d.s. for 14 days (see BNF 2019); IV: 25–50 mg/kg daily or 1–2 g in 6 even doses (eMC 11/1/2018)

Route of admin
Oral, IV

Contraindications
Hypersensitivity, hepatic dysfunction

Side effects
Nausea, vomiting, diarrhoea, fever, skin eruptions, urticaria, rashes, cardiac arrhythmias; in large doses – reversible hearing loss, hepatic dysfunction, thrombophlebitis following IV administration, allergic response rare with mild anaphylaxis

Interactions
Anticoagulants – effect of warfarin enhanced
Antihistamines – inhibits the metabolism of terfenadine, causing dangerous cardiac arrhythmias
Cisapride – can cause cardiotoxicity and arrhythmias
Ergotamines – acute ergot toxicity, rapid peripheral vasospasm and dysaesthesia
Theophylline – inhibition of metabolism of theophylline

Pharmacodynamic properties
Antimicrobial that attaches to a subunit of susceptible organisms and suppresses protein synthesis, destroying cell wall stability and making them vulnerable to attack. Active against both Gram-positive and Gram-negative bacteria, mycoplasms, treponema, chlamydia and gonorrhoea

Fetal risk
Crosses the placental barrier but not in appreciable quantities; fetal concentrations have found to be low, with no reports of congenital defects located except in animal studies – cardiovascular malformations if used in early pregnancy. However, manufacturers advise that, if used to treat maternal syphilitic infection during pregnancy, the infant may be born with congenital syphilis and should receive penicillin treatment following birth

Breastfeeding
Secreted in only small amounts in breast milk – considered safe with no ill effects reported, although manufacturers advise avoidance

BP
Cefuroxime

Proprietary
Cefuroxime (Sandoz Ltd)
Cefuroxime (Bowmed Ibisque Ltd)
Zinicef (GlaxoSmithKline UK)
Cefuroxime (non-proprietary, see BNF for details)

Group
Antibiotic – cephalosporin

Uses/indications
Against both Gram-positive and Gram-negative bacteria, prophylaxis with LSCS, UTI, respiratory infections

Type of drug
POM

Presentation
Capsules, syrup, powder for reconstitution

Dosage
Oral: 250–500 mg b.d. or 0.5–1 g b.d. (eMC 2/8/2016)
IM, IV: 500 mg–1 g q.d.s. given over 3–5 min, max 3–6 g per day for severe infections e.g. gonorrhoea or meningitis (eMC 13/3/2018)

Route of admin
Oral, IM, IV

Contraindications
Renal dysfunction, known hypersensitivity to cephalosporins, caution in penicillin hypersensitivity

Side effects
Nausea, diarrhoea and hypersensitivity – usually mild, headache, dizziness, dyspnoea

Interactions
Nil specific to cephradine:
Anticoagulants – effect of warfarin enhanced
Uricosurics – excretion is reduced by probenecid
Oestrogens – reduces the effect of the combined oral contraceptive pill

Pharmacodynamic properties
Broad-spectrum bactericidal drug active against
Gram-positive organisms, e.g. staphylococci, streptococci, *Streptococcus pyogenes, Streptococcus pneumoniae,* and Gram-negative organisms such as *Escherichia
coli, Haemophilus influenzae,* salmonella. Highly active
against penicillinase-producing staphylococci. e.g.
Staphylococcus aureus

Fetal risk
Cefuroxime has been shown to cross the placenta and
attain therapeutic levels in amniotic fluid and cord
blood after intramuscular or intravenous dose to the
mother

Breastfeeding
Excreted in human milk in small quantities. Adverse
reactions at therapeutic doses are not expected

BP
Flucloxacillin sodium

Proprietary
Flucloxacillin (Aurobinda Pharma-Milpharm Ltd)
Flucloxacillin powder for injection or infusion
(Wockhardt UK Ltd)
Flucloxacillin (non-proprietary, see BNF for details)

Group
Antibiotic, penicillinase-resistant penicillin

Uses/indications
Against β-lactamase Gram-positive resistant microbes,
including *S. aureus* and streptococci; prophylaxis in
surgery

Type of drug
POM

Continued

Presentation
Capsules, syrup, powder for reconstitution

Dosage
Oral: 250–500 mg t.d.s. (30–60 min before food) (eMC 3/1/2018)
IV/infusion: 250 mg–2 g q.d.s. (eMC 12/1/2018)
IM: 250–500 mg q.d.s. (according to severity of infection) (eMC 12/1/2018)
Prophylaxis: 1–2 g IV at induction of anaesthesia, then 500 mg q.d.s. IM or IV for up to 72 hours (eMC 12/1/2018)

Route of admin
Oral, IM, IV/infusion

Contraindications
Penicillin and/or cephalosporin hypersensitivity, sodium-restricted diet, renal or hepatic impairment

Side effects
Anaphylaxis – uncommon and usually mild and transitory, diarrhoea, rash, indigestion, rarely hepatic impairment, reversible neutropenia, thrombocytopenia

Interactions
Contraceptives – reduces contraceptive effect

Pharmacodynamic properties
Narrow-spectrum penicillin that is not inactivated by staphylococcal lactamases. It acts on the synthesis of the bacterial wall and exerts a bactericidal effect on streptococci, including *Neisseria* and *Clostridia,* but not MRSA

Fetal risk
Animal studies show no teratogenicity but manufacturer advises that it should be withheld unless considered essential

Breastfeeding
Trace quantities can be detected in breast milk; considered safe, but as for amoxicillin

BP
Co-amoxiclav (compound of Amoxicillin as a sodium salt and Clavulanic acid)

Proprietary
Augmentin (GlaxoSmithKline UK)
Augmentin for infusion (GlaxoSmithKline UK)
Co-amoxiclav (non-proprietary, see BNF for details)

Group
Antibiotic, broad-spectrum penicillinase

Uses/indications
Against bacteria resistant to amoxicillin, i.e. *S. aureus, E. coli,* gonorrhoea, β-lactamase infection, UTI, abdominal infection, cellulitis, prophylaxis at LSCS or MRP

Type of drug
POM

Presentation
Tablets, dispersible tablets, suspension, powder for reconstitution

Dosage
Oral: 375 mg (250 mg expressed as amoxicillin plus 125 mg of clavulanic acid) t.d.s.; 625 mg (500 mg) t.d.s in severe infection (eMC 7/3/2018)
IV: 600 mg–1.2 g t.d.s. (eMC 7/3/2018) max 3 g per day

Route of admin
Oral, IV, IV infusion

Contraindications
Penicillin and/or cephalosporin hypersensitivity, jaundice/hepatic dysfunction

Side effects
Nausea, diarrhoea, rashes, rarely hepatic impairment, hypersensitivity, CNS effects – rare, vaginal itching, soreness and discharge

Continued

Interactions
Nil specific
Anticoagulants – may prolong bleeding time and
prothrombin time
Contraceptives – reduces contraceptive effect

Pharmacodynamic properties
Resistance to antibiotics is caused by bacterial
enzymes destroying it before it is able to act on the
pathogen. The clavulanate anticipates this and blocks
β-lactamase enzymes in organisms sensitive to amoxicillin. Co-amoxiclav has a rapid bactericidal effect

Fetal risk
Animal studies with oral and parenteral administration show no teratogenicity, but manufacturers advise
avoidance in the first trimester and use thereafter only
when considered essential; second/third trimesters – a
single study of women with preterm premature rupture of membranes given Augmentin for prophylaxis
against infection found an association with necrotiz-
ing enterocolitis in the neonate (SPmC – Augmentin®
GlaxoSmithKline UK 07/03/18)

Breastfeeding
Little known of effects of clavulanic acid on breastfed
infants; trace quantities of amoxicillin excreted but
considered safe – as for amoxicillin

BP
Amoxicillin trihydrate or sodium

Proprietary
Amoxicillin capsules (Aurobindo Pharma-Milpharm Ltd)
Amoxicillin powder for solution for injection vials
(Bowmed Ibisqus Ltd)
Amoxicillin (non-proprietary, see BNF for details)

Group
Antibiotic, broad-spectrum penicillinase

Uses/indications
Broad spectrum; used against aerobes Gram-positive, e.g. *Streptococcus*, *Staphylococcus* and *Listerisa monocytogenes* and Gram-negative bacteria, e.g. *Haemophilus influenza*, *Escherichia coli* and *Salmonella* species, except *Pseudomonas*, and anaerobes, e.g. *Closteridium*; also respiratory infections, UTI, gonorrhoea, puerperal sepsis

Type of drug
POM

Presentation
Capsules, dispersible tablets, suspension – paediatric and adult, powder for reconstitution

Dosage
Oral: 250–500 mg t.d.s. (eMC 18/10/2017)
IM: 500 mg t.d.s.
IV: 500 mg t.d.s. to 1 g q.d.s. in severe infection (eMC 7/12/2017)
Prophylaxis: 1 g IV, then 500 mg 6 hours later (eMC 7/12/2017)

Route of admin
Oral, IM, IV/infusion

Contraindications
Penicillin hypersensitivity

Side effects
Mild diarrhoea, indigestion, rash, rarely anaphylaxis – usually mild

Interactions
Anticoagulants – causes prolonged prothrombin time
Contraceptives – reduces contraceptive effect
Uricosurics – excretion reduced with concomitant administration of probenecid – used in treatment of gonorrhoea

Continued

Pharmacodynamic properties
Broad-spectrum antibiotic with rapid bactericidal effects; which has the safety profile of penicillin

Fetal risk
Nil known, no reports of toxicity in animal or human studies, but manufacturers advise benefits should outweigh the risks

Breastfeeding
Considered safe but modifies the bowel flora and can cause sensitizaton; interferes with culture results if an infection screen is required

---

BP
Trimethoprim

Proprietary
Co-trimoxazole (Accord-UK Ltd)
Trimethoprim (Accord-UK Ltd)
Trimethoprim (non-proprietary, see BNF for details)

Group
Antimicrobial – sulphonamide

Uses/indications
Treatment of sensitive organisms, UTI, URTI, prophylaxis against UTI

Type of drug
POM

Presentation
Tablets, suspension, injection

Dosage
Oral: 2 tablets or 100–200 mg b.d.
IV injection/infusion: 200 mg b.d.
Prophylaxis: 100 mg daily (eMC 7/7/2018)

Route of admin
Oral, IV

Contraindications
Pregnancy, hypersensitivity to trimethoprim, blood dyscrasias, renal insufficiency or impairment

Side effects
Nausea, vomiting, rash – mild and reversible, allergic reactions, including anaphylaxis

Interactions
Anticonvulsants – half-life of phenytoin is increased, antifolate effect enhanced
Anticoagulants – enhanced anticoagulant effect
Oestrogens – reduces the effect of the combined oral contraceptive pill

Pharmacodynamic properties
Antimicrobial that works by selective inhibition of bacterial dihydrofolate reductase. It is effective against both Gram-positive and Gram-negative aerobic organisms, including *E. coli, Proteus, Klebsiella, S. aureus, Streptococcus. faecalis* and *pneumoniae, Haemophilus influenzae,* but NOT *Neisseria, Pseudomonas aeruginosa, Treponema pallidum* or anaerobes

Fetal risk
First trimester: teratogen – as a folate antagonist, manufacturers advise avoidance as can cause transient hyperbilirubinaemia in the neonate (Weiner and Mason, 2017)

Breastfeeding
Excreted in small amounts but considered moderately safe in the short term

BP
Gentamicin sulfate

Proprietary
Gentamicin injection (Hospira UK Ltd)
Cidomycin solution for injection (SANOFI)
Gentamicin (non-proprietary, see BNF for details)

Group
Broad-spectrum aminoglycoside antibiotic

Uses/indications
Gram-positive and Gram-negative pathogens, systemic infection, prophylaxis during labour for patients with heart valves/heart disease, UTI, chest infection

Type of drug
POM

Presentation
Ampoules

Dosage
IM or slow IV injection: 3–5 mg/kg body weight daily in divided doses, e.g. 80 mg 8 hourly in patients over 60 kg, or 60 mg 8 hourly in those under 60 kg (eMC 8/5/2018)

Route of admin
IM, IV slow injection, IV infusion

Contraindications
Hypersensitivity, myasthenia gravis, renal impairment

Side effects
Toxicity – renal toxicity reversible after withdrawal. Vestibular hearing loss/damage, hypersensitivity

Interactions
Avoid concomitant use with ototoxic and nephrotoxic drugs
Muscle relaxants – enhances the muscle relaxant effect
Oestrogens – may reduce the effect of the combined oral contraceptive pill

Pharmacodynamic properties
Bactericidal aminoglycoside that acts by inhibiting protein synthesis, acting on the integrity of the plasma membrane and metabolism of ribonucleic acid

Fetal risk
Safety is not established and it crosses the placental barrier second/third trimester – probably low risk but potentially may cause deafness

Breastfeeding
Present in breast milk, and although unlikely to cause problems the manufacturers advise avoidance

---

BP
Benzylpenicillin sodium

Proprietary
Benzylpenicillin sodium powder for injection (Genus Pharmaceuticals)
Benzylpenicillin sodium (non-proprietary, see BNF for details)

Group
Antibiotic – penicillinase

Uses/indications
Streptococcal infection, i.e. throat infection, ear infection, pneumonia, treatment of gonorrhoea

Type of drug
POM

Presentation
Vials of powder for reconstitution

Dosage
IM, IV injection or IV infusion: 600 mg to 3.6 g in four divided doses (available in 600 mg and 1200 mg doses equivalent to 1 and 2 mega units) (eMC 16/9/2016)

Continued

Route of admin
IM, IV injection/infusion

Contraindications
Hypersensitivity to penicillin

Side effects
Hypersensitivity – urticaria, fever, joint pain, rashes, anaphylaxis, diarrhoea, thrombocytopenia, neutropenia, haemolytic anaemia – in high doses

Interactions
Nil specific
Oestrogens – reduces the effect of combined oral contraceptive pill

Pharmacodynamic properties
Bacteriostatic with bactericidal activities against Gram-negative coli. It is inactivated by gastric acid and is therefore best given IV or by injection

Fetal risk
Nil reported

Breastfeeding
It is not known if benzylpenicillin sodium may be excreted into the breast milk of nursing mothers although other penicillins have been detected

BP
Ampicillin trihydrate

Proprietary
Penbritin (Chemidex Pharma Ltd)
Ampicillin powder for injection (AAH Pharmaceuticals Ltd)
Ampicillin (non-proprietary, see BNF for details)
Also as mix of ampicillin sodium and flucloxacillin sodium – Magnapen powder for solution for injection or infusion (Wockhardt UK Ltd)

Group
Broad-spectrum antibiotic, penicillin

Uses/indications
Wide range of bacterial infections including UTI, ear infection, sinusitis, bronchitis, *Haemophilus influenzae,* salmonella, meningococcal disease, listerial meningitis

Type of drug
POM

Presentation
Capsules, suspension, vials for injection

Dosage
Oral: 0.25–1 g q.d.s. (taken 30 min before food) (eMC 5/1/2016)
IM, IV/IVI: 500 mg 4–6 hourly (see BNF 2019)

Route of admin
Oral, IM, IV

Contraindications
Hypersensitivity to penicillin, history of renal impairment, caution with erythematous rash

Side effects
Gastrointestinal disturbances, rashes, hypersensitivity – anaphylaxis

Interactions
Antibiotics – concurrent use of bacteriostatic drugs can interfere with the bactericidal action of ampicillin
Anticoagulants – INR may be altered by course of broad-spectrum antibiotics
Oestrogens – reduces the effectiveness of combined oral contraceptive pill

Pharmacodynamic properties
Broad-spectrum antibiotic indicated in the treatment of a wide range of bacterial infections caused by ampicillin-sensitive organisms

Continued

Fetal risk

Manufacturer advises documentary evidence of clinical use in pregnancy extensively since 1961 with no shown teratogenic effects

Breastfeeding

Trace amounts excreted into breast milk, but there are no adequate data about use during lactation; no advice regarding avoidance

References and Recommended Reading

Ampicillin 500mg powder for solution for injection or infusion. Last updated on the BNF [online] October 2019.

Beigi, R. (2015). The importance of studying antimicrobials in pregnancy. *Seminars in perinatology*, *39*, 556–560.

Berlin, C. (2013). Medications and the breastfeeding mother. In D. Mattison (Ed.), *Clinical pharmacology during pregnancy* (pp. 41–54). Edinburgh: Elsevier.

Briggs, G., Freeman, R., Towers, C., & Forinash, A. (2017). *Drugs in pregnancy and lactation: A reference guide to fetal and neonatal risk* (11th ed.). Philadelphia: Wolters Kluwer.

Fisher, B., & Yudin, M. (2017). Other infectious conditions in pregnancy. In D. James, P. Steer, P. ,C. Weiner, B. Gonik, & S. Robson (Eds.), *High risk pregnancy: Management options* (5th ed.) (pp. 729–778). Cambridge: Cambridge University Press.

Furber, C., Allison, D., & Hindley, C. (2017). Antimicrobial resistance, antibiotic stewardship, and the role of the midwife's role. *British Journal of Midwifery*, *25*(11), 693–698.

MBRRACE–UK. (2018). MBRRACE-UK: *Saving Lives, Improving Mothers' Care. Lessons learned to inform maternity care from the UK and Ireland. Confidential Enquiries into Maternal Deaths and Morbidity 2014–16* Oxford: MBRRACE/NPEU. Available from: https://www.npeu.ox.ac.uk/mbrrace-uk/reports. [Accessed 12 April 2019].

National Institute for Health and Care Excellence (NICE). (2008). CG 64 *Prophylaxis against infective endocarditis: Antimicrobial prophylaxis against infective endocarditis in adults and children undergoing interventional procedures* [online]. Last updated July 2016. London: NICE. Available from: https://www.nice.org.uk/guidance/cg64 Pathway

Available from: http://pathways.nice.org.uk/pathways/prophylaxis-against-infective-endocarditis. [Accessed 12 June 2019].

National Institute for Health and Care Excellence (NICE). (2008). *CG 70 Inducing labour* [online]. Last updated January 2017. London: NICE. Available from https://www.nice.org.uk/guidance/cg70. [Accessed 22 June 2019].

National Institute for Health and Care Excellence (NICE). (2012). *CG 149 Neonatal infection (early onset): Antibiotics for prevention and treatment* [online]. Last updated January 2017. London: NICE. Available from https://www.nice.org.uk/guidance/cg149. [Accessed 22 June 2019].

National Institute for Health and Care Excellence (NICE). (2015). *NG 5 Medicines optimisation: The safe and effective use of medicines to enable the best possible outcomes* [online]. Last updated March 2019. London: NICE. Available from https://www.nice.org.uk/guidance/ng5. [Accessed 16 April 2019].

National Institute for Health and Care Excellence (NICE). (2015). *NG 25 Preterm labour and birth* [online]. Last updated January 2017. London: NICE. Available from https://www.nice.org.uk/guidance/ng25. [Accessed 22 June 2019].

National Institute for Health and Care Excellence (NICE). (2016). *NG 51 Sepsis: Recognition, diagnosis and early management.* Last updated September 2017. London: NICE. Available from https://www.nice.org.uk/guidance/ng51. [Accessed 12 June 2019].

National Institute for Health and Care Excellence (NICE) and Public Health England (PHE). (2019). *Summary of antimicrobial prescribing guidance – managing common infections.* London: NMC. Available from https://www.nmc.org.uk/globalassets/sitedocuments/standards/standards-of-proficiency-for-midwives.pdf. [Accessed 20 November 2019].

Nursing and Midwifery Council (NMC), 2019. *Standards of proficiency for midwives.* London: NICE. Available from https://www.nice.org.uk/Media/Default/About/what-we-do/NICE-guidance/antimicrobial%20guidance/summary-antimicrobial-prescribing-guidance.pdf. [Accessed 12 June 2019].

Royal College of Obstetricians and Gynaecologists (RCOG). (2012). *GTG 64b Sepsis following Pregnancy, Bacterial* [online]. London: RCOG. Available from https://www.rcog.org.uk/globalassets/documents/guidelines/gtg_64b.pdf. [Accessed 12 June 2019].

Royal College of Obstetricians and Gynaecologists (RCOG). (2012). *GTG 64a Sepsis in Pregnancy, Bacterial* [online]. London: RCOG. Available from https://www.rcog.org.uk/globalassets/documents/guidelines/gtg_64a.pdf. [Accessed 12 June 2019].

Royal College of Obstetricians and Gynaecologists (RCOG). (2017). *GTG 36 Prevention of Early Onset Neonatal Group B Streptococcal Disease* [online]. London: RCOG. Available from https://obgyn.onlinelibrary.wiley.com/doi/full/10.1111/1471-0528.14821. [Accessed 22 June 2019].

Royal College of Obstetricians and Gynaecologists (RCOG). (2019). *GTG 73 Care of Women Presenting with Suspected Preterm Prelabour Rupture of Membranes from 24⁺⁰ Weeks of Gestation* [online]. London: RCOG. Available from https://obgyn.onlinelibrary.wiley.com/doi/10.1111/1471-0528.15803. [Accessed 22 June 2019].

Royal Pharmaceutical Society and Royal College of Nursing. (2019). *Professional Guidance for the Administration of Medicines in Healthcare Settings. Endorsed by RCM*. London: RPS.

SmPC from the eMC. Amoxicillin 250mg and 500mg capsules. Aurobindo Pharma-Milpharm Ltd. Last updated on the eMC 18/10/2017.

SmPC from the eMC. Amoxicillin 250mg and 500mg powder for solution for injection vials. Bowmed Ibisqus Ltd. Last updated on the eMC 07/12/2017.

SmPC from the eMC. Augmentin® 375mg tablets and Augmentin® intravenous injection. GlaxoSmithKline Ltd. Last updated on the eMC 07/03/2018.

SmPC from the eMC. Benzylpenicillin sodium 600mg and 1.2g powder for injection. Genus Pharmaceuticals. Last updated on the eMC 16/09/2016.

SmPC from the eMC. Cefuroxime 250mg tablets. Sandoz Ltd. Last updated on the eMC 02/08/2016.

SmPC from the eMC. Cefuroxime 250mg powder for injection. Bowmed Ibisqus Ltd. Last updated on the eMC 13/03/2018.

SmPC from the eMC. Cidomycin 80mg/2mL solution for injection. SANOFI. Last updated on the eMC 21/01/2019.

SmPC from the eMC. Co-trimazole® 80mg/400mg tablets. Accord-UK Ltd. Last updated on the eMC 25/07/2018.

SmPC from the eMC. Erythrocin 250mg and 500mg tablets. ADVANZ Pharma. Last updated on the eMC 14/02/2018.

SmPC from the eMC. Erythromycin 1g powder for solution for injection. ADVANZ Pharma. Last updated on the eMC 11/1/2018.

SmPC from the eMC. Flagyl® 200mg tablets. SANOFI. Last updated on the eMC 18/10/2018.

SmPC from the eMC. Flagyl® 400 mg tablets, and 500 mg suppositories. SANOFI. Last updated on the eMC 23/10/2018.

SmPC from the eMC. Flucloxacillin 250mg and 500mg capsules. Aurobindo Pharma-Milpharm Ltd. Last updated on the eMC 03/01/2018.

SmPC from the eMC. Flucloxacillin 250mg and 500mg Powder for solution for injection or infusion. Wockhardt UK Ltd. Last updated on the eMC 12/01/2018.

SmPC from the eMC. Gentamicin 40 mg/ml injection. Hospira UK Ltd. Last updated on the eMC 08/05/2018.

SmPC from the eMC. Magnapen® 250mg/250mg powder for solution for injection or infusion. Wockhardt UK Ltd. Last updated on the eMC 22/04/2016.

SmPC from the eMC. Metronidazole 500 mg/100 ml for intravenous infusion. Baxter Healthcare Ltd. Last updated on the eMC 11/02/2018.

SmPC from the eMC. Penbritin® 250mg and 500mg capsules. Chemidex Pharma Ltd. Last updated on the eMC 05/01/2016.

SmPC from the eMC. Trimethoprim® 200mg tablets. Accord-UK Ltd. Last updated on the eMC 07/07/2018.

SmPC from the eMC. Zinacef® 250mg, 75-mg and 1.5g powder for injection. GlaxoSmithKline Ltd. Last updated on the eMC 01/02/2019.

Tomlinson, M. (2017). Cardiac disease in pregnancy. In D. James, P. Steer, C. Weiner, B. Gonik, & S. Robson (Eds.), *High risk pregnancy: Management options* (5th ed.) (pp. 900–943). Cambridge: Cambridge University Press.

Tutt, M., & Jordan, S. (2010). Antimicrobial agents. In S. Jordan (Ed.), *Pharmacology for midwives: The evidence base for safe practice* (2nd ed.) (pp. 284–307). Basingstoke: Palgrave Macmillan.

Weiner, C., Gotsch, F., & Romero, R. (2017). Intrauterine infection, preterm parturition, and the fetal inflammatory response syndrome. In D. James, P. Steer, P. ,C. Weiner, B. Gonik, & S. Robson (Eds.), *High risk pregnancy: Management options* (5th ed.) (pp. 597–603). Cambridge: Cambridge University Press.

Weiner, C., & Mason, C. (2017). Medication. In D. James, P. Steer, C. Weiner, B. Gonik, & S. Robson (Eds.), *High risk pregnancy: Management options* (5th ed.) (pp. 808–846). Cambridge: Cambridge University Press.

Further Reading

Macdonald, S., & Johnson, G. (2017). *Mayes' midwifery* (15th ed.). Edinburgh: Elsevier.

Marshall, J., & Raynor, M. (Eds.). (2014). *Myles textbook for midwives* (16th ed.) Edinburgh: Churchill Livingstone.

5

Anticoagulants

Anticoagulants are substances used to prevent blood clotting.
The student should be aware of:

- factors predisposing to thromboembolism
- local protocols for management of thromboembolism
- the antagonist for such treatment and its availability
- factors involved in the mechanism of blood clotting, and the criteria used to determine which is the most appropriate anticoagulant
- conditions requiring treatment with anticoagulants
- maternal and fetal sequelae of such treatment
- the effects of progesterone on the circulatory system.

Heparin antagonist: protamine sulphate
Warfarin antagonist: vitamin K and plasma

BP
Heparin (as sodium or calcium salt)

Proprietary
Heparin Sodium (Panpharma UK Ltd)
Clexane pre-filled syringes (enoxaparin sodium) (SANOFI)
Fragmin single dose syringe (delteparin sodium)
(Pfizer Ltd)

Group
Anticoagulant, parenteral

Uses/indications
Treatment of DVT, pulmonary embolism, thrombo-embolism – susceptible clients, prophylaxis in LSCS or high risk due to impaired mobility

Type of drug
POM

Presentation
Preloaded syringes, vials

Dosage
Prophylactic and/or during pregnancy: 5–10 000 units b.d. – haematological monitoring required (see BNF 2019)

For DVT – IV: 5000 units loading dose and then continuous infusion of 15–25 units/kg/hour adjusted by laboratory monitoring (severe PE: loading dose 10 000 units), followed by 15,000 units b.d (see BNF 2019)

S.C.: after LSCS 4000 units high risk until ambulant; 2000 units for moderate risk for 6–14 days (eMC 28/2/2018)

NB Benzyl alcohol (preservative) crosses placenta so manufacturers recommend use preparation without preservative.

Route of admin
S.C., IV

Contraindications
Haemorrhagic disorders, including heparin-induced thrombocytopenia, cerebral aneurysm, cerebral vascular accident/cerebral haemorrhage, severe hypertension, peptic ulcer, haemophilia, liver disease, major trauma, hypersensitivity, threatened abortion

Side effects
Haemorrhage, including placental sites, thrombocytopenia hypersensitivity, bruising and haematoma formation. Prolonged use is associated with osteoporosis

Continued

Interactions

Nil specific

Anticoagulants – concomitant use enhances effects: use caution when transferring to oral anticoagulants

Antihistamines – decreases the anticoagulant effect

Aspirin – antiplatelet effect enhanced by heparin

Diclofenac – increased risk of haemorrhage (with IV diclofenac)

GTN – the excretion of heparin is increased by the GTN decreasing the anticoagulant effect

NSAIDs IV – possible increased risk of bleeding

Pharmacodynamic properties

A naturally occurring anticoagulant that is synthesized and excreted by mast cells in the body. It acts by forming a complex with antithrombin, catalysing the inhibition of several activated blood coagulation factors and thrombin. This prevents the conversion of fibrinogen to fibrin, which is crucial for clot formation. The onset of action is immediate; and it is most commonly used for the prevention and treatment of venous and arterial thromboembolism

Fetal risk

Available data suggest there is no risk to fetus or neonate

Breastfeeding

Not excreted in breast milk

NB: discontinue use prior to epidural anaesthesia, i.e. 8–12 hours; can cause spinal haematoma or permanent paralysis

OVERDOSE Indicated by haemorrhage; APTT and platelet count should be determined. Minor haemorrhage rarely requires specific treatment; and decreasing or delaying subsequent doses of heparin should be sufficient. Major haemorrhage: the anticoagulant

effect is reduced immediately by 1% protamine
sulphate, but caution is required as protamine also has
an anticoagulant effect. A single dose should never
exceed 50 mg IV injection of protamine can cause a
sudden fall in blood pressure, bradycardia, dyspnoea
and transitory flushing, but this can be avoided or
decreased by slow and careful administration

BP
Warfarin sodium

Proprietary
Warfarin (Ranbaxy [UK] Limited, a Sun Pharmaceutical
Company)
Warfarin sodium (non-proprietary, see BNF for details)

Group
Anticoagulant – oral

Uses/indications
Prophylaxis after prosthetic heart valve surgery, DVT,
pulmonary embolism, and transient ischaemic attacks

Type of drug
POM

Presentation
Tablets, white 0.5 mg, brown 1 mg, blue 3 mg, pink
5 mg

Dosage
Refer to pharmacist or BNF; usually 3–10 mg daily
tailored to individual requirements. Baseline prothrombin measurements (PT) should be taken before
beginning therapy with warfarin (eMC 24/5/2017)

Route of admin
Oral

Continued

Contraindications

Pregnancy, but may be used between 16 and 36 weeks' gestation if heparin not available and risks of thrombosis outweigh the risk to the fetus; peptic ulcer, severe hypertension, bacterial endocarditis, haemorrhage; use within 24 hours of surgery or labour – caution if needed

Side effects

Haemorrhage, nausea, transient alopecia, hypersensitivity, fall in haematocrit value, purple toes, liver dysfunction, pancreatitis

Interactions

Alcohol – enhanced effects with large alcohol doses

Antacids – cimetidine inhibits the metabolism and enhances the effect of warfarin

Aspirin – increased risk of haemorrhage – antiplatelet effect

Antibiotics – cephalosporins, macrolides, erythromycin and metronidazole, sulphonamides, trimethoprim – possible enhanced coagulant effect

Penicillins – possible alteration of INR

Antidepressants – SSRIs – anticoagulant effect increased

Dextropropoxyphene – anticoagulant effect enhanced

Paracetamol – theoretical increased risk of bleeds with prolonged use

Cholestyramine – enhanced anticoagulant effect

Barbiturates – metabolism of warfarin increased, therefore diminishes the anticoagulant effect

Antiepileptics – carbamazepine and phenobarbital – diminishes the anticoagulant effect

Phenytoin – both enhances and diminishes warfarin's effect

Sodium valproate – enhanced anticoagulant effect

Oral contraceptive – diminished contraceptive effect

NSAIDs – enhanced anticoagulant effect

Mefenamic acid – enhances anticoagulant effect

Progestogen – antagonism of anticoagulant effect

Pharmacodynamic properties

Synthetic anticoagulant of the coumarin series. It acts by inhibiting the formation of active clotting factors II, VII, IX and X. An effective prothrombin time (PT) can be achieved in 24–36 hours post initial dose, max 36–48 hours, and this therapeutic PT is maintained for 48 hours after stopping drug

Fetal risk

Fetal teratogen, causes multiple disorders and malformations; should be stopped preconception or within 6 weeks' gestation (see contraindications above); haemorrhage in fetus and placenta in all trimesters; postnatal developmental delay

Breastfeeding

Excreted in breast milk in small amounts; theoretical risk of haemorrhage, especially with vitamin K deficiency, but considered safe if dose within therapeutic range

New medications being marketed that have similar pharmacotherapeutic properties to warfarin sodium are:

- Pradaxa (dabigatran etexilate mesilate) (Boehringer Ingelheim Ltd)
- Xarelto (rivaraxaban) (Bayer PLC).

These drugs require less frequent monitoring of clotting times. Currently there is no indication of their efficacy or safety during childbearing.

BP
Protamine sulfate

Proprietary
Prosulf (Wockhardt UK Ltd)
Protamine sulfate (AAH Pharmaceuticals Ltd)
Protamine sulfate (non-proprietary, see BNF for detail)

Continued

Group
Heparin antagonist

Uses/indications
Reversal of the actions of heparin

Type of drug
POM

Presentation
Ampoules

Dosage
See BNF and manufacturers' guidelines. *In brief:* 1 mg neutralizes 100 units heparin (mucus) or 80 units (lung) within 15 min of administration; if longer, less is required as heparin is rapidly excreted. Max dose 50 mg in 10 min. Should be monitored by activated partial prothrombin time (APPT) or other clotting test 5–10 min after administration; further doses may be required as protamine is cleared more rapidly than heparin, especially LMWH (eMC 9/5/2018)

Route of admin
Slow IV injection

Contraindications
Hypersensitivity to protamine; caution in those receiving protamine insulin preparation, i.e. isophane insulin, fish allergy

Side effects
Flushing, nausea, vomiting, hypotension, bradycardia; if overdosed then acts as an anticoagulant

Interactions
Caution in those receiving *isophane insulins* – hypersensitivity

Pharmacodynamic properties
A potent antidote to heparin but the precise mechanism is unknown. It is assumed that the strongly basic protamine combines with the strongly acid heparin to produce a stable salt that has no anticoagulant activity

Fetal risk
Insufficient information available – no animal or human studies have been carried out

Breastfeeding
No data available – as for fetal risk

BP
Phytomenadione (Vitamin K)

Proprietary
Konakion MM 10 mg in 1 mL and Konakion MM Paediatric 2 mg in 0.2 mL (Cheplapharm Arzneimittel GmbH)

Group
Warfarin antagonist

Uses/indications
Prevention and treatment of haemorrhage

Type of drug
POM, Midwives' Exemption (paediatic dose only)

Presentation
Ampoules

Dosage

Refer to manufacturers' guidelines:
Adult: Prophylaxis – *Obstetric cholestasis and epilepsy;* from 36 weeks of pregnancy (RCOG, 2011 and 2016 respectively) recommend 10 mg daily especially when APPT is prolonged, or if steatorrhoea is present (eMC 3/4/2019)
Life-threatening haemorrhage: 5 mg slow IV injection plus plasma

Continued

(factors II, IX, VII if available)

Less severe haemorrhage: withhold warfarin and consider 0.5–2 mg slow IV injection repeat APPT levels 3 hours post dose and if not responsive then repeat dose – not more than 40 mg in 24 hours (eMC 3/4/2019)

Paediatric: *Prophylaxis – Vitamin K deficiency bleeding: Healthy newborns of 36 weeks' gestation and older:*
Either 1 mg administered by IM injection at birth or soon after birth **or** 2 mg orally at birth or soon after birth. The oral dose should be followed by a second dose of 2 mg at 4–7 days

Exclusively breast-fed babies who received oral Konakion at birth: In addition to the doses at birth and at 4–7 days, a further 2 mg oral dose should be given 1 month after birth

Pre-term neonates of less than 36 weeks' gestation weighing 2.5 kg or more, and term neonates at special risk: 1 mg IM or IV at birth or soon after birth, the size and frequency of further doses depending on coagulation status

Pre-term neonates of less than 36 weeks' gestation weighing less than 2.5 kg: 0.4 mg/kg (equivalent to 0.04 mL/kg) IM or IV at birth or soon after birth (eMC 3/4/2019). The frequency of further doses should depend on coagulation status

Haemorrhage: initial dose of 1 mg IV and further dose will depend on coagulation profile

Route of admin
Very slow IV injection, oral, IM

Contraindications
No data available

Side effects
Anaphylactoid reactions after intravenous injections of Konakion MM; rarely, venous irritation or phlebitis

Interactions
Anticoagulants – antagonism of the anticoagulant effect

Pharmacodynamic properties
Synthetic vitamin K. Vitamin K is essential for the formation of prothrombin, factor VII, factor IX, and factor X. Without vitamin K there is a tendency to haemorrhage

Fetal risk
Poor placental transfer; no risk data available

Breastfeeding
Maternal doses – not enough information available to allow classification as safe drug. Large maternal doses of anticoagulants may require neonatal vitamin K prophylaxis

Low molecular weight heparin (LMWH) acts slightly differently to unfractionated heparin (UFH). It is essential to have an understanding of the coagulation cascade in order to understand how and why heparin is an anticoagulant. The advantage of LMWH over UFH is in its action: the actions of UFH are influenced by its binding to plasma protein, endothelial cell surfaces, macrophages and other acute-phase reactants in the anticoagulant cascade. LMWH has decreased binding to non-anticoagulant-related plasma proteins. The anticoagulant response is predictable and reproducible, with no need for laboratory monitoring, and it is given on a weight-adjusted basis. It has a high bioavailability of 90%, compared with 30% for UFH, and has a longer plasma half-life of 4–6 hours versus 0.5–1 hours for UFH. There is less inhibition of platelet function and potentially less bleeding risk, although this is unproven. There is a lower incidence of thrombocytopenia and thrombosis as there is less interaction with platelet factor 4 (Hirsch et al., 2001; Available from: https://pdfs.semanticscholar.org/b6b9/253a96b5f9f8ade3a8412799a0f69c306108.pdf).

The next three examples are some of the LMWH and their dosages, properties, pregnancy and breastfeeding risks:

■ OVERDOSE: protamine sulphate only partially neutralizes these drugs, so use with caution and consider the side effects of protamine carefully.

BP
Dalteparin sodium

Proprietary
Fragmin (Pfizer Ltd)

Group
LMWH

Presentation
Single-dose syringe, ampoules, vials

Dosage
PE/DVT: S.C., depending on body weight: 69–82 kg, 15 000 units daily; 83 kg and over, 18 000 units daily; oral anticoagulants can be used concomitantly until therapeutic range is achieved (usually 5 days) (eMC 19/5/2016)

Route of admin
S.C.

Pharmacodynamic properties
Porcine-derived sodium heparin and antithrombotic agent with the ability to potentiate the inhibition of Factor Xa and thrombin by antithrombin. This ability is relatively higher than disruption of the plasma clotting line (expressed as APTT); therefore, compared with UFH, dalteparin has fewer adverse effects on platelet function and adhesion, thus giving only minimal effects on primary haemostasis

Fetal risk
Does not pass the placenta; as for heparin

Breastfeeding
As for heparin

BP
Enoxoparin

Proprietary
Clexane (SANOFI)
Enoxaparin sodium (non-proprietary, see BNF for details)

Group
LMWH

Presentation
Single-dose syringe, vials

Dosage
PE/DVT: S.C. 1.5 mg/kg every 24 hours for at least 5 days or until oral anticoagulation is established (150 units/kg daily)
NB: unlicensed indication for use during pregnancy for treatment of venous thromboembolism. Prophylaxis: moderate risk 20 mg (2000 units) daily for 7–10 days
High risk: 40 mg (4000 units) daily for 6 days or until ambulant

Route of admin
S.C.

Pharmacodynamic properties
LMWH with antithrombotic activity. There is a greater rate of this than with UFH, and at the recommended dose it does not significantly alter platelet aggregation, the binding of fibrinogen to platelets, or global clotting tests such as APTT and PT time

Fetal risk
No evidence that enoxaparin crosses the placental barrier; evidence of risk in the second trimester but no information on the first and third trimesters. As there are no adequate controlled studies it is not advised for use unless there is no safe alternative

Breastfeeding
Excretion into breast milk is unlikely but manufacturer advises avoidance

BP
Tinzeparin sodium

Proprietary
Innohep (Leo Laboratories Ltd)
Tinzeparin sodium (Alliance Healthcare Ltd)

Group
LMWH

Presentation
Single-dose syringe, ampoules

Dosage
Caution: can cause bronchospasm and shock in asthmatics
PE/DVT: S.C. 175 units/kg daily for 6 days or until oral anticoagulation is established after epidural/spinal anaesthesia; delay subsequent dose by at least 4 hours

Route of admin
S.C.

Pharmacodynamic properties
Antithrombotic agent that acts by inhibiting the action of several activated coagulation factors, especially Factor Xa

Fetal risk
No transplacental transmission has been found in the second trimester, but studies in rats show low birthweight; therefore the manufacturer advises avoidance

Breastfeeding
No evidence of excretion found, but manufacturer advises avoidance

References and Recommended Reading

Berlin, C. (2013). Medications and the breastfeeding mother. In D. Mattison (Ed.), *Clinical pharmacology during pregnancy* (pp. 41–54). Edinburgh: Elsevier.

Eliott, D., & Pavord, S. (2013). Thrombo-embolic disorders. In E. Robson, & J. Waugh (Eds.), *Medical disorders in pregnancy: A manual for midwives* (2nd ed.) (pp. 279–298). Chichester, WSussex: Wiley Blackwell.

Gilbert, E. (2011). *Venous thromboembolic disease. Manual of high risk pregnancy and delivery* (5th ed.). St Louis: Mosby/Elsevier, 282–288.

Herbert, M. (2013). Impact of pregnancy on maternal pharmacokinetics of medications. In D. Mattison (Ed.), *Clinical pharmacology during pregnancy* (pp 17–40). Edinburgh: Elsevier.

Hirsh, J., Warkentin, T., Shaughnessy, S., Anand, S., Halperin, J., Raschke, R., Granger, C., Ohman, E., & Dalen, J. (2001). Heparin and low-molecular-weight heparin. mechanisms of action, pharmacokinetics, dosing, monitoring, efficacy, and safety. *Chest, 119* (1 Suppl), 64S–94S.

Johnson, R., & Taylor, W. (2016). *Skills for midwifery practice* (4th ed.). Edinburgh: Elsevier.

Jordan, S. (2010). Drugs affecting the coagulation process. In S. Jordan (Ed.), *Pharmacology for Midwives: The evidence base for safe practice* (2nd ed.) (pp. 199–220). Basingstoke: Palgrave Macmillan.

Jordan, S., & MacDonald, S. (2017). Pharmacology and the midwife. In S. MacDonald, & G. Johnson (Eds.), *Mayes' Midwifery: A text book for midwives* (15th ed.) (pp. 158–174). Edinburgh: Elsevier.

MBRRACE–UK, (2018). MBRRACE-UK: *Saving Lives, Improving Mothers' Care. Lessons learned to inform maternity care from the UK and Ireland. Confidential Enquiries into Maternal Deaths and Morbidity 2014–16.* Oxford: MBRRACE/NPEU. Available from: https://www.npeu.ox.ac.uk/mbrrace-uk/reports. [Accessed 12 April 2019].

National Institute of Health and Care Excellence (NICE). (2011). *CG132. Caesarean section* [online]. Last updated August 2012. London: NICE. Available from: https://www.nice.org.uk/guidance/cg132. [Accessed 14 April 2019].

National Institute of Health and Care Excellence (NICE). (2006). *CG37. Postnatal care up to 8 weeks after birth* [online]. Last updated February 2015. London: NICE. Available from: https://www.nice.org.uk/guidance/cg37.[Accessed 14 April 2019].

Nursing and Midwifery Council (NMC), (2019). *Standards of proficiency for midwives.* London: NMC. Available from: https://www.nmc.org.uk/globalassets/sitedocuments/standards/standards-of-proficiency-for-midwives.pdf. [Accessed 20 November 2019].

Rang, H., Ritter, J., Flower, R., & Henderson, G. (2016). *Rang and Dale's pharmacology* (8th ed.). Edinburgh: Elsevier Churchill Livingstone.

Rankin, J. (2017). Anaemia and clotting disorders. In J. Rankin (Ed.), *Physiology in childbearing with anatomy and related biosciences* (pp. 343–352). Edinburgh: Elsevier.

Royal College of Obstetricians and Gynaecologists. (2015). *GTG 37a Reducing the Risk of Venous Thromboembolism during Pregnancy and the Puerperium*. London: RCOG. Available from: https://www.rcog.org.uk/globalassets/documents/guidelines/gtg-37a.pdf. [Accessed 22 May 2019].

Royal College of Obstetricians and Gynaecologists. (2015). *GTG 37b Thromboembolism during Pregnancy and the Puerperium: Acute Management*. London: RCOG. Available from: https://www.rcog.org.uk/globalassets/documents/guidelines/gtg-37b.pdf. [Accessed 22 May 2019].

SmPC from the eMC. Clexane® 2,000 units, 4,000 units, 6,000 units, 8,000 units and 10,000 units in solution for injection in pre-filled syringes. SANOFI. Last updated on the eMC 20/9/2018.

SmPC from the eMC. Fragmin® 5,000 unit pre-filled syringes. Pfizer Ltd. Last updated on the eMC 19/5/2016.

SmPC from the eMC. Heparin 5,000 iu/mL solution for injection (without preservative). Panpharma UK Ltd. Last updated on the eMC 28/2/2018.

SmPC from the eMC. innohep® 10,000 iu/mL in pre-filled syringes. Leo Laboratories Ltd. Last updated on the eMC 30/3/2017.

SmPC from the eMC. Konakion® 10mg/mL for injection. Cheplapharm Arzneimittel GmbH. Last updated on the eMC 3/4/2019.

SmPC from the eMC. Konakion® 2mg/0.2mL for injection. Cheplapharm Arzneimittel GmbH. Last updated on the eMC 3/4/2019.

SmPC from the eMC. Pradaxa® 75mg capsules. Boehringer Ingelheim Ltd. Last updated on the eMC 26/2/2018.

SmPC from the eMC. Prosulf® 10mg/mL solution for injection. Wockhardt UK Ltd. Last updated on the eMC 9/5/2018.

SmPC from the eMC. Warfarin 0.5mg, 1mg, 3mg and 5mg tablets. Ranbaxy (UK) Limited, a Sun Pharmaceutical Company. Last updated on the eMC 24/5/2017.

SmPC from the eMC. Xarelto® 2.5mg tablets. Bayer PLC. Last updated on the eMC 29/8/2018.

Weiner, C., & Mason, C. (2017). Medication. In D. James, P. Steer, C. Weiner, B. Gonik, & S. Robson (Eds.), *High risk pregnancy: Management options* (5th ed.) (pp. 808–846). Cambridge: Cambridge University Press.

Further Reading

Phytomenadione for newborns. See https://bnfc.nice.org.uk/drug/phytomenadione.html [Accessed 22 May 2019].

6

Antiepileptic Medication

Anticonvulsants are drugs used to arrest or prevent fits or seizures. The benefits of treatment should outweigh the risk to the fetus, and efforts should be made to use the single most effective drug, as teratogenicity increases with the number of drugs used. Pre-conceptual advice is strongly recommended (see latest advice on Sodium Valporate on GOV.UK 2018, NICE 2019).

This drug group inhibits the uptake of folic acid, and therefore any supplements given may need to be continued throughout pregnancy.

Magnesium sulfate is also an anticonvulsant used in the emergency treatment of eclampsia – see Chapter 15.

The student should be aware of:

- conditions that require anticonvulsant therapy
- local protocols for anticonvulsant therapy and specific medical conditions
- recognition of fits, seizures and convulsions
- resuscitative techniques and care of affected clients
- maternal and fetal sequelae of absorption of these preparations.

Interactions

Phenytoin

Alcohol – high intake increases plasma phenytoin levels; chronic abuse decreases serum levels

Analgesics – NSAIDs increase the plasma phenytoin concentration

Antacids – reduce the absorption of phenytoin; cimetidine decreases the metabolism of phenytoin and therefore increases its plasma concentration

Antibiotics – metronidazole increases the plasma phenytoin concentration; plasma concentration and antifolate effect increased by co-trimoxazole and trimethoprim

Anticoagulants – probably reduce the effect of warfarin

Antidepressants – tricyclics decrease the phenytoin plasma concentration and the convulsive threshold

Antiepileptics – two or more antiepileptics enhance toxicity; monitoring of plasma concentrations required

Antiemetics – stemetil and derivatives lower convulsive threshold

Antihypertensives – nifedipine increases phenytoin plasma concentration; the effect of nifedipine is reduced

Anxiolytics and hypnotics – diazepam can increase or decrease plasma phenytoin concentration

Corticosteroids – metabolism is increased, so effect is decreased

Contraceptives – metabolism of oral contraceptives is increased, so their effect is decreased

Vitamins – the plasma phenytoin concentration is lowered by folic acid; vitamin D supplements may be required.

Phenobarbital

Alcohol – increased sedative effect

Antibiotics – metabolism of metronidazole is increased, so the effect is decreased

Anticoagulants – metabolism of warfarin increased, so effect is decreased

Antidepressants – tricyclics decrease the plasma concentration and the convulsive threshold

Antiepileptics – as for phenytoin; requires dose monitoring

Antiemetics – as for phenytoin

Antihypertensives – effect of nifedipine reduced

Corticosteroids – as for phenytoin

Contraceptives – as for phenytoin

Folic acid – phenobarbital has antifolate effect

Sodium valproate

Analgesics – aspirin enhances effect

Antacids – cimetidine increases plasma levels of valproate

Antibiotics – erythromycin increases plasma levels of valproate

Anticoagulants – increased anticoagulant effect – monitoring of PT required

Antiemetics – as for phenytoin

Antiepileptics – with two or more, close monitoring is required

Cholestyramine – decreases absorption of valproate

Zidovudine – antagonism of the metabolism of zidovudine, so increased toxicity

Carbamazepine

Alcohol – enhanced CNS effects

Anticoagulants – decreased anticoagulant effect of warfarin

Antidepressants – tricyclics have an accelerated metabolism, so decreased effect; monitoring required

Antiepileptics – plasma concentration effected by concomitant use, so careful plasma monitoring required

Cimetidine – inhibits the metabolism of carbamazepine, so increases plasma concentration

Corticosteroids – carbamazepine increases the metabolism of both β-prednisolone and dexamethasone

Dextropropoxyphene – increases effect of carbamazepine

Erythromycin – increased plasma concentrations of carbamazepine

Nifedipine – decreased antiepileptic effect

OCP – decreased contraceptive effect

Tramadol – decreased effect of tramadol

BP
Phenytoin

Proprietary
Epanutin (Pfizer Ltd)
Phenytoin (Aurobindo Pharma – Milipharm Ltd)
Phenytoin (non-proprietary, see BNF for details)

Group
Anticonvulsant/antiepileptic

Uses/indications
Epilepsy, fits – not absence seizures, treatment of eclampsia

Type of drug
POM

Presentation
Capsules, tablets, suspension

Dosage
Initial dose 3–4 mg/kg/day with or after food: maintenance doses 200–500 mg/day in 1–2 divided doses or as per protocol (plasma values need evaluation and adjustment) (eMC 1/11/2018)
IV: phenytoin sodium in treatment of status epilepticus as per protocol, e.g. 20 mg/kg (max. per dose 2 g), then (by intravenous infusion or by slow intravenous injection or by mouth) maintenance 100 mg every 6–8 hours adjusted according to plasma-concentration monitoring

Route of admin
Oral, IV

Contraindications
Pregnancy and breastfeeding, hepatic impairment, hypersensitivity, shock

Side effects
OVERDOSE: no known antidote – possibly removed from plasma by haemodialysis
Nausea, vomiting, headache, tremor, insomnia; prolonged usage – hirsutism, coarse facies, acne, gingival hyperplasia, confusion

Interactions
See start of chapter

Pharmacodynamic properties
Appears to stabilize rather than raise seizure threshold, and to prevent the spread of seizure activity rather than abolish the primary focus of seizure discharge. The mechanism is not fully understood but may include:
• a reduction in sodium conductance by enhancing its extrusion, thereby preventing potential seizure activity
• enhancing the action of GABA inhibition and reducing excitatory synaptic transmission
• presynaptic reduction of calcium entry and block of release of neurotransmitters

Fetal risk
Know teratogen in trimesters 1 and 3; maternal folic acid supplements should be given under medical supervision; increased risk of haemorrhage in the neonate – prophylaxis with vitamin K recommended

Breastfeeding
Secreted in breast milk, some minor effects noted, mother and child should be monitored, manufacturer advises avoidance unless necessary

BP
Phenobarbital

Proprietary
Phenobarbital (Accord-UK Ltd)
Phenobarbital (non-proprietary, see BNF for details)

Group
Antiepileptic – barbiturate

Uses/indications
Epilepsy – not absence seizures

Type of drug
POM, CD

Presentation
Tablets, solution and solution for injection

Dosage
Oral: 60–180 mg at night (monitoring for plasma-phenobarbital concentration for optimum response is 15–40 mg/litre (60–180 micromol/litre) (eMC 13/2/2019); however, monitoring the plasma-drug concentration is less useful than with other drugs because tolerance occurs)
Status epilepticus: 10 mg/kg by injection (max. per dose 1 g), dose to be administered at a rate not more than 100 mg/minute, injection to be diluted 1 in 10 with water for injections (eMC 13/2/2018)

Route of admin
Oral, IM, IV injection

Contraindications
Pregnancy, breastfeeding, impaired hepatic or renal function, respiratory depression

Side effects
Tolerance develops, drowsiness, neural depression, allergic skin reactions, overdose

Interactions
See start of chapter

Pharmacodynamic properties
A long-acting barbiturate that is an effective anti-convulsant. It appears to raise/elevate the seizure threshold and limit the spread of seizure activity. The mechanism is unknown but may involve an increase in the GABA synergic systems

Fetal risk
In trimesters 1 and 3, a teratogen, particularly neural tube defects, hypoprothrombinaemia and withdrawal in infants with maternal treatment late in pregnancy; concomitant administration with other antiepileptics has been linked to haemorrhagic disease of the newborn within the first 24 hours of life – prophylaxis with vitamin K is recommended

Breastfeeding
Avoid where possible, as drowsiness in infant and other minor effects reported. Mother and baby need to be monitored

BP
Carbamazepine

Proprietary
Tegretol (Novartis Pharmaceuticals UK Ltd)
Carbamazepine (non-proprietary, see BNF for details)

Group
Anticonvulsant

Uses/indications
Epilepsy, generalized seizures and partial seizures, not absence seizures or myoclonic seizures (trigeminal neuralgia)

Type of drug
POM

Presentation
Tablets, suppositories, liquid, chewtabs

Dosage
Oral: initially 100–200 mg 1–2 times a day, increased in steps of 100–200 mg every 2 weeks; usual dose 0.8–1.2 g daily in divided doses; increased if necessary up to 1.6–2 g daily in divided doses (eMC 12/4/2019)

P.R.: Up to 1 g daily in 4 divided doses for up to 7 days, for short-term use when oral therapy temporarily not possible

Route of admin
Oral, P.R.

Contraindications
Pregnancy, breastfeeding, history of bone marrow depression, hepatic/renal impairment, blood hepatic or skin disorders, glaucoma, sensitivity to either carbamazepine or structurally similar drugs, use of tricyclic or MAOI drugs

Side effects
Side effects are common and appear dose related, resolving spontaneously or after transient dose reduction; gastrointestinal disturbances, drowsiness, headaches, visual disturbances, rashes, blood disorders, including thrombocytopenia, hepatic/renal disorders

Interactions
See start of chapter

Pharmacodynamic properties
Exact mechanism unknown, but thought to stabilize hyperexcited nerve membranes, inhibiting repetitive neuronal discharges and reducing excitatory impulses. It also reduces glutamate release and blockades sodium channels, thereby stabilizing neuronal membranes and action potentials

Fetal risk

Animal studies show an increase in mortality if taken during organogenesis; later administration caused growth retardation in rat fetuses – women who take carbamazepine should be counselled for risk and given antenatal screening, and the benefits of administration should be weighed against the risks. There is also a theoretical risk of HDN in the neonate, therefore prophylactic vitamin K is recommended

Breastfeeding

Excreted but considered safe in common doses, although manufacturer recommends observation for side effects

The following medication Sodium Valproate has been contraindicated in the UK for use with women/girls of childbearing potential (GOV.UK 2018, NICE 2019).

BP

Sodium valproate, valproic acid (https://www.gov.uk/government/news/valproate-banned-without-the-pregnancy-prevention-programme)

Proprietary

Epilim (SANOFI)
Sodium valproate (non-proprietary, see BNF for details)

Group

Anticonvulsant

Uses/indications

All forms of epilepsy

Type of drug

POM

Presentation

Tablets, solution, syrup, powder for reconstitution

Continued

Dosage
Oral: 600 mg–2.5 g/day in two divided doses titrated against body weight (eMC 18/12/2018)
IV/IV infusion: same as oral but over 3–5 min (eMC 7/2/2019)

Route of admin
Oral, IV/IV infusion

Contraindications
Valproate is no longer prescribed to women/girls of childbearing potential (GOV.UK 2018, NICE 2019), pregnancy and breastfeeding, hepatic or renal impairment, SLE

Side effects
Gastrointestinal disturbances, nausea, ataxia, tremor, weight gain, hair loss, hepatic impairment, disturbed platelet function, pancreatitis; multiple therapy requires care

Interactions
See start of chapter

Pharmacodynamic properties
Likely mode of action is potentiation of the inhibitory action of GABA, through action on the further synthesis or metabolism of GABA

Fetal risk
Spina bifida, neonatal bleeding, hepatotoxicity, fetal growth deficiency, hyperbilirubinaemia, fetal distress, craniofacial defects, urogenital defects, hypospadias up to 50%, retarded psychomotor development, digital abnormalities

Breastfeeding
Secreted in breast milk – in low doses appears safe; high doses – insufficient information to qualify as safe

References and Recommended Reading

Berlin, C. (2013). Medications and the breastfeeding mother. In D. Mattison (Ed.), *Clinical Pharmacology During Pregnancy* (pp. 41–54). Edinburgh: Elsevier.

Briggs, G., Freeman, R., Towers, C., & Forinash, A. (2017). *Drugs in Pregnancy and Lactation: a reference guide to fetal and neonatal risk* (11th ed.). Philadelphia: Wolters Kluwer.

Carbamazepine 125mg suppositories AAH Pharmaceuticals Ltd. Last updated on the BNF [online] April 2019.

Carhuapoma, J., Varner, M., & Levine, S. (2017). Neurologic Complications in Pregnancy. In D. James, P. Steer, C. Weiner, B. Gonik, & S. Robson (Eds.), *High Risk Pregnancy: Management options* (5th ed.) (pp. 1273–1321). Cambridge: Cambridge University Press.

UK, G. O. V. (2018). *Guidance Valproate use by women and girls.* [online] Available from: https://www.gov.uk/guidance/valproate-use-by-women-and-girls. [Accessed 4 July 2019].

Herbert, M. (2013). Impact of pregnancy on maternal pharmacokinetics of medications. In D. Mattison (Ed.), *Clinical Pharmacology During Pregnancy* (pp. 17–40). Edinburgh: Elsevier.

Jordan, S., & MacDonald, S. (2017). Pharmacology and the midwife. In s. MacDonald, & G. Johnson (Eds.), *Mayes' Midwifery: A Text Book for Midwives* (15th ed.) (pp. 158–174). Edinburgh: Elsevier.

MBRRACE–UK. (2018). *MBRRACE-UK: Saving Lives, Improving Mothers' Care. Lessons learned to inform maternity care from the UK and Ireland. Confidential Enquiries into Maternal Deaths and Morbidity 2014–16.* Oxford: MBRRACE/NPEU. Available from: https://www.npeu.ox.ac.uk/mbrrace-uk/reports. [Accessed 12 April 2019].

McAuliffe, F., Burns-Kent, E., Frost, D., & Howarth, E. (2013). Neurological disorders. In E. Robson, & J. Waugh (Eds.), *Medical Disorders in Pregnancy: A Manual for Midwives* (2nd ed.) (pp. 125–152). Chichester, WSussex: Wiley Blackwell.

National Institute for Health and Care Excellence (NICE). (2019). Sodium Valporate. Available from https://bnf.nice.org.uk/drug/sodium-valproate.html#importantSafetyInformations. [Accessed 4 July 2019].

Nursing and Midwifery Council (NMC). (2019). *Standards of proficiency for midwives.* London: NMC. Available from: https://www.nmc.org.uk/globalassets/sitedocuments/standards/standards-of-proficiency-for-midwives.pdf. [Accessed 20 November 2019].

Royal College of Obstetrics and Gynaecology. (2016). *GTG 68 Epilepsy in pregnancy*. London: RCOG. Available from: https://www.rcog.org.uk/globalassets/documents/guidelines/green-top-guidelines/gtg68_epilepsy.pdf. [Accessed 22 May 2019].

Sassarini, J., Clerk, N., & Jordan, S. (2010). Epilepsy in pregnancy. In S. D. Jordan (Ed.), *Pharmacology for Midwives: The Evidence Base for Safe Practice* (2nd ed.) (pp. 361–376). Basingstoke: Palgrave Macmillan.

SmPC from the eMC. Epanutin infatabs 50 mg tablets. Pfizer Limited. Last updated on the eMC 29/5/2019.

SmPC from the eMC. Epilim® 200mg tablets. SANOFI. Last updated on the eMC 18/12/2018.

SmPC from the eMC. Phenytoin 100mg tablets. Aurobindo Pharma - Milpharm Ltd. Last updated on the eMC 1/11/2018.

SmPC from the eMC. Phenytoin injection. Hospira UK Ltd. Last updated on the eMC 15/8/2017.

SmPC from the eMC. Phenobarbital 60mg tablets. Accord-UK Ltd. Last updated on the eMC 13/2/2019.

SmPC from the eMC. Phenobarbital Sodium 60mg/mL injection. Martindale Pharma. Last updated on the eMC 23/1/2018.

SmPC from the eMC. Sodium Valproate 100mg/mL solution for injection or infusion. Wockhardt UK Ltd. Last updated on the eMC 7/2/2019.

SmPC from the eMC. Tegretol® 100mg and 200mg tablets. Novartis Pharmaceuticals UK Ltd. Last updated on the eMC 12/4/2019.

SmPC from the eMC. Tegretol® 100 mg/5mL liquid. Novartis Pharmaceuticals UK Ltd. Last updated on the eMC 11/4/2019.

Weiner, C., & &Mason, C. (2017). Medication. In D. James, P. Steer, C. Weiner, B. Gonik, & S. Robson (Eds.), *High Risk Pregnancy: Management Options* (5th ed.) (pp. 808–846). Cambridge: Cambridge University Press.

7

Antidepressants and Treatments for Mental Health Conditions

Midwives will encounter women with enduring mental health disorders as well as women who develop a range of varied illnesses during the childbearing continuum. Specialist care pathways and collaborative psychiatric services are essential to support maternity care and essential management of pharmacotherapeutic regimes. Two of the commonest medicine groups are antidepressants and antipsychotics.

Antidepressants

These are preparations that aim to restore the balance of neurotransmitter substances in the brain, a deficiency of which is thought to contribute to depression. They are usually selective serotonin reuptake inhibitors (SSRIs), monoamine oxidase inhibitors (MAOIs) or tricyclic antidepressants.

St John's wort (*Hypericum perforatum*) is a popular herbal remedy for mild depression. However, it does interact with many prescribed medications including antidepressants, and its use should be carefully monitored and advice sought from a medical practitioner.

Antimania or Antipsychotic Drugs

These are medications used to control acute and episodes of mania or hypomania. Benzodiazepines are also used to treat behavioural disturbances.

The licensed use of valproate in epilepsy and also in bipolar disorder for the management mania or hypomania for women with childbearing potential is not recommended by the MHRA and NICE (GOV.UK 2018 and NICE 2019). This is due to significant risk of malformations and developmental abnormalities associated with taking valproate during pregnancy (see reference for NICE 2019).

The student should be aware of:

- the possible biological, psychological and sociological causative factors which contribute to emotional processing difficulties for women especially during childbearing
- the role of the midwife in early risk assessment and interprofessional collaboration for women with enduring and childbirth related mental health conditions
- the clinical signs and progression of antenatal and postnatal depression (PND)
- the maternal and fetal sequelae of therapy
- the local availability of counselling and facilities for treatment
- the consequences for lack of either diagnosis or treatment of mental health issues
- the research into PND and its relation to hypothyroidism in certain cases.

CAUTION: The authors recommend that drugs in this group should be investigated individually, as psychiatry is a specialised field and most antidepressants and antipsychotic medicines require comprehensive monitoring in pregnancy, labour, postnatal periods and during breastfeeding.

Tricyclic Antidepressants (TCA)

BP
Dosulepin hydrochloride

Proprietary
Prothiaden (Teofarma)
Dosulepin hydrochloride (AAH Pharmaceuticals Ltd)
Dosulepin hydrochloride (non-proprietary, see BNF for details)

Group
Antidepressant – tricyclic

Uses/indications
Depression where sedation is required, e.g. postnatal depression

Type of drug
POM

Presentation
Capsules (25 mg), tablets (75 mg)

Dosage
Oral: 75 mg daily (divided doses, titrated to symptoms using a stepped approach for increase/decrease) increased to 150–225 mg daily (maintenance) (see BNF 2019)

Route of admin
Oral

Contraindications
Recent myocardial infarction, mania

Side effects
Dry mouth, sedation, blurred vision, cardiovascular disturbances, blood sugar changes

Interactions
Alcohol – avoid – enhanced sedative effect
Antidepressants – CNS excitation, hypertension with MAOIs – avoid for 2 weeks after stopping MAOI

Continued

Antiepileptics – convulsive threshold and tricyclic plasma concentration are lowered

Antihistamines – increased antimuscarinic and sedative effect, ventricular arrhythmias with terfenadine and astemizole

Antihypertensives – increases hypotensive effect

Contraceptives – antagonizes effect of antidepressants, but side effects increase the plasma concentration of tricyclics

Pharmacodynamic properties

Tricyclic antidepressant that acts to increase transmitter levels at central synapses; this produces a clinical antidepressant effect. The inhibition of the re-uptake of noradrenaline (norepinephrine) and 5-hydroxytryptamine (5HT) and the uptake of dopamine produces adaptive changes in the brain that enhance the antidepressant effects

Fetal risk

Higher fetal toxicity than SSRIs; tachycardia, irritability, muscle spasms and neonatal convulsions

Breastfeeding

Amount secreted too small to be harmful in short-term use; accumulation may cause sedation and respiratory depression

Other tricyclic antidepressants which block the re-uptake of serotonin or noradrenaline:

Clomipramine hydrochloride
Imipramine hydrochloride
Amitriptyline hydrochloride
Doxepin hydrochloride
Lofepramine hydrochloride
Nortriptyline hydrochloride
Trimipramine maleate

Selective Serotonin Reuptake Inhibitor Antidepressants (SSRIs)

BP
Fluoxetine

Proprietary
Prozac (Eli Lilly & Co. Ltd)
Fluoxetine (Accord Healthcare Ltd)
Fluoxetine (non-proprietary, see BNF for details)

Group
Antidepressant – SSRI

Uses/indications
Depressive illness, bulimia nervosa, obsessive–compulsive disorder

Type of drug
POM

Presentation
Tablets (10 mg) or capsules (20 or 60 mg), dispersible tablets, liquid (5 mL = 20 mg)

Dosage
20 mg daily (varies according to condition, max 60 mg) (eMC 9/3/2017 and 14/5/2018)
Long half-life
Cessation of therapy: Withdrawal will occur within 5 days, and medical support and advice should be available. The dose should be tapered over at least a few weeks to avoid effects such as gastrointestinal disturbances, headache, anxiety, dizziness, paraesthesia, electric shock sensation in the head, neck, and spine, tinnitus, sleep disturbances, fatigue, influenza-like symptoms, and sweating. Most symptoms will be mild and self-limiting, but can be severe.

Continued

Route of admin

Oral

Contraindications

Mania, cardiac disease, epilepsy, hepatic/renal impairment, pregnancy, breastfeeding, concomitant use of MAOI

Side effects

Gastrointestinal disturbances, hypersensitivity, anxiety, palpitations, tremors, hair loss, confusion, hypotension, drowsiness, blood disorders, liver disturbances, suicidal thoughts

Seratonin syndrome – excessive serotonergic agonism within CNS, thought to be due to noradrenergic hyperactivity, and mediation probably due to 5-HT_{2A} receptor agonism. Treatment depends on severity including reduce/withdraw medication, may need intubation if severe reaction

Interactions

Alcohol – alcohol and SSRIs are inadvisable
Antidepressants – enhance toxicity and levels require monitoring
Antiepileptics – carbamazepine and phenytoin enhance toxicity and levels require monitoring
Anticoagulants – warfarin – increased bleeding time, levels need monitoring
Antihypertensives – enhanced hypotensive effect

Pharmacodynamic properties

Selective inhibitor of serotonin reuptake

Fetal risk

First trimester – cardiovascular anomalies; third trimester – risk (5 per 1000 pregnancies) of persistent pulmonary hypertension in the newborn (PPHN); manufacturer advises use only if the benefits outweigh the risks post-birth: these effects have been reported in neonates – irritability, tremor, hypotonia, persistent crying, difficulty in sucking or in sleeping

Breastfeeding

Significant amounts are excreted into milk as the metabolite norfluoxetine; manufacturer advises avoidance unless the benefits outweigh the risks and the lowest dose of medication is used

Other SSRI medications

Citalopram hydrochloride/hydrobromide
Dapoxetine hydrochloride
Escitalopram oxalate
Fluvoxamine maleate
Paroxetine hydrochloride
Sertraline hydrochloride
Selective inhibition of the re-uptake of serotonin (5-hydroxytryptamine, 5-HT).

Noradrenaline reuptake inhibitor or Serotonin and Noradrenaline Reuptake Inhibitor (NRI or SNRIs)

Bupropion hydrochloride
Duloxetine hydrochloride
Naltrexone hydrochloride
Venlafaxine hydrochloride
Inhibition of the re-uptake of serotonin and/or noradrenaline

Other antidepressant medications – MAOI group

Medications include: Isocarboxazid, Phenelzine (Nardil), or Tranylcypromine
MAOIs inhibit monoamine oxidase, thereby causing an accumulation of amine neurotransmitters.
Increased risk of neonatal malformations – manufacturer advises avoid unless there are compelling reasons.
Avoid during breastfeeding.

BP
Progesterone

Proprietary
Cyclogest (LD Collins &Co Ltd)
Progesterone (non-proprietary, see BNF for details)

Group
Hormones – progesterone

Uses/indications
Premenstrual syndrome, puerperal depression – although there is no convincing evidence of physiological effectiveness, may be used for the alleviation of PND

Type of drug
POM

Presentation
Off-white pessaries (for vaginal or rectal use)

Dosage
200–400 mg once or twice a day (eMC 28/9/2018)

Route of admin
P.R., P.V.

Contraindications
Diabetes, breastfeeding, hypertension, renal, hepatic or cardiac disease

Side effects
Acne, urticaria, fluid retention, weight change, gastro-intestinal disturbances, changes in libido

Interactions
None known

Pharmacodynamic properties
Progestational steroid

Fetal risk
High doses can be teratogenic in the first trimester
Manufacturers recommend Cyclogest should not be used during pregnancy

Breastfeeding
High doses can inhibit or suppress lactation
Manufacturers recommend Cyclogest should not be
used during breastfeeding

BP
Lithium carbonate/Lithium citrate

Proprietary
Priadel (lithium carbonate) (SANOFI)
Priadel Liquid (lithium citrate) (SANOFI)
Lithium carbonate or citrate (non-proprietary, see BNF
for details)

Group
Antimania drug

Uses/indications
Management of acute manic or hypomanic episodes,
recurrent depressive disorders where treatment with
other antidepressants has been unsuccessful, prophylaxis for bipolar affective disorders, control of aggres-
sive behaviour or intentional self-harm

Type of drug
POM

Presentation
(Prolonged release) tablet, liquid

Dosage
Priadel® prolonged release tablets 400–1200 mg in
single dose, morning or before bed in addition, doses
can be divided as b.d. (eMC 20/9/2018)
CAUTION: regular monitoring of serum lithium
levels, monitoring of well-being and planned multi-
professional care plans are recommended in providing
care for women on lithium medications (NICE 2014)

Route of admin
Oral

Contraindications

Diabetes, untreated hypothyroidism, breastfeeding, hypertension, renal, hepatic or cardiac disease

Side effects

Acne, urticaria, fluid retention, weight change, gastro-intestinal disturbances, changes in libido

Interactions

Antibiotics – reduce renal clearance, e.g. metronidazole, tetracyclines, co-trimazole, trimethoprim

ACE inhibitors, diuretics, NSAIDs, steroids – increase lithium concentrations (risk of toxicity). *Sodium-based products, caffeine, theophylline, diuretics, urea* – decrease lithium concentrations

Antipsychotics (clozapine, haloperidol), carbamazepine, phenytoin, methyldopa, tricyclic antidepressants, calcium channel blockers, SSRIs, NSAIDs – neurotoxicity, even if lithium levels in normal range

NB: lithium toxicity can also occur when other health issues arise, e.g. infection, pregnancy-onset conditions, physical or psychological changes

Pharmacodynamic properties

Mood-stabilizing agent; lithium is an alkali metal as lithium carbonate or lithium citrate; modifies the production and turnover of certain neurotransmitters, particularly serotonin, and may also block dopamine receptors; modifies concentrations of some electrolytes, particularly calcium and magnesium; and may reduce thyroid activity

Fetal risk

High doses can be teratogenic in the first trimester – cardiac anomalies especially. Ebstein anomaly, and other malformations have been reported. Neonates may show signs of lithium toxicity including symptoms such as lethargy, flaccid muscle tone, or hypotonia.

Breastfeeding

Is secreted in breast milk and there have been case reports of neonates showing signs of lithium toxicity

BP
Methadone

Proprietary
Methadone (Martindale Pharma)
Methadone (non-proprietary, see BNF for details)

Group
Substance dependence

Uses/indications
Management of opioid dependence under the supervision of an appropriate physician or pharmacist for community support

Type of drug
POM

Presentation
Clear or light green solution for oral use

Dosage
Calculated for individual and serum monitoring. Initially 10–20 mg/day, increasing by 10–20 mg daily until there is no sign of withdrawal or intoxication. The usual dose is 40–60 mg/day (eMC 31/10/2019). Drug withdrawal needs to be achieved 4–6 weeks before delivery if neonatal abstinence syndrome is to be certain to be avoided, but abrupt withdrawal can cause intrauterine death. Detoxification to abstinence is least stressful to mother and fetus if undertaken during the mid-trimester (eMC 31/10/2019)
NB: long half-life in system

Route of admin
Oral – not for dilution or injection unless specified by manufacturer

Continued

Contraindications

Hypersensitivity, acute asthma, head injury, acute alcoholism, concurrent use of MAOIs **Pregnancy/ labour** – not recommended as may cause neonatal respiratory depression, withdrawal symptoms in the neonate Manufacturers advise caution in hypothyroidism, adrenal disease, inflammatory bowel disease

Side effects

Overdose: symptoms/signs in methadone overdose are essentially as for morphine, although methadone has a greater respiratory depressive effect and a lesser sedative effect than an equivalent dose of morphine

Toxicity: highly variable dosages, regular use leading to tolerance. Pulmonary oedema is a common effect of overdose; dose-related histamine-releasing property of methadone may cause urticaria and pruritus; may lead to an increase in intracranial pressure

Interactions

Naloxone (opioid antagonist) – counteracts the effects of methadone and induces abstinence. **CNS depressants** – may result in increased respiratory depression, hypotension, strong sedation or coma. Slow tolerance development; every dose increase may after 1–2 weeks give rise to symptoms of respiratory depression. Dose adjustments must be monitored carefully

Peristalsis inhibition – e.g. loperamide and methadone may result in severe constipation and increase the CNS depressant effects

Antidepressants (paroxetine, sertraline) or antibiotics (erythromycin, clarithromycin) – may cause changes to cardiac contractility (QT)

MAOIs – CNS inhibition, serious hypotonia and/or apnoea 2 weeks after cessation of treatment **Opioid analgesics** – delay gastric emptying.

Pharmacodynamic properties

Methadone is an opioid analgesic similar to morphine and is highly addictive; less sedative effect than morphine. It acts on the CNS system and smooth muscle via specific opiate receptor sites in the brain, spinal cord and nervous system Methadone is an opioid agonist with actions predominantly at the μ receptor

Fetal risk

Limited data in humans show no increased risk of congenital abnormalities

Withdrawal symptoms/respiratory depression may occur in neonates of mothers treated with methadone chronically during pregnancy. Generally advisable not to detoxify the patient, especially starting this process after the 20th week of pregnancy, but to administer maintenance treatment with methadone. Methadone should be withheld just before and during birth because of the risk of neonatal respiratory depression

Breastfeeding

Excreted in breast milk; average breast-milk/plasma ratio is 0.8 for measures in μg/mL for methadone concentrations; manufacturer recommends the benefits must be weighed against the risks to the infant

References and Recommended Reading

Berlin, C. (2013). Medications and the breastfeeding mother. In D. Mattison (Ed.), *Clinical pharmacology during pregnancy* (pp. 41–54). Edinburgh: Elsevier.

Briggs, G., Freeman, R., Towers, C., & Forinash, A. (2017). *Drugs in pregnancy and lactation: A reference guide to fetal and neonatal risk* (11th ed.). Philadelphia: Wolters Kluwer.

Di Mambro, B. (2017). Mental health disorders in pregnancy. In D. James, P. Steer, C. Weiner, B. Gonik, & S. Robson (Eds.), *High risk pregnancy: Management options* (5th ed.) (pp. 1501–1522). Cambridge: Cambridge University Press.

Dosulepin hydrochloride 25mg capsules or 75mg tablets.

AAH Pharmaceuticals Ltd. Last updated on the BNF [online] April 2019.

GOV.UK, (2018). *Guidance Valproate use by women and girls.* [online] Available from: https://www.gov.uk/guidance/valproate-use-by-women-and-girls. [Accessed 4 July 2019].

Gutteridge, K. (2017). Maternal mental health and psychological issues. In S. Macdonald, & G. Johnson (Eds.), *Mayes' midwifery* (15th ed.) (pp. 1130–1147). Edinburgh: Elsevier.

Herbert, M. (2013). Impact of pregnancy on maternal pharmacokinetics of medications. In D. Mattison (Ed.), *Clinical pharmacology during pregnancy* (pp. 17–40). Edinburgh: Elsevier.

Jordan, S., & Hardy, B. (2010). Drugs and mental health. In S. Jordan (Ed.), *Pharmacology for midwives: The evidence base for safe practice* (2nd ed.) (pp. 377–394). Basingstoke: Palgrave Macmillan.

LaRusso, E., & Freeman, M. (2013). Antidepressants in pregnancy. In D. Mattison (Ed.), *Clinical pharmacology during pregnancy* (pp. 295–306). Edinburgh: Elsevier.

Lazerus, R., & Gutteridge, K. (2013). Psychiatric disorders. In E. Robson, & J. Waugh (Eds.), *Medical disorders in pregnancy: A manual for midwives* (2nd ed.) (pp. 319–332). Chichester, WSussex: Wiley Blackwell.

MBRRACE–UK. (2018). MBRRACE-UK: *Saving Lives, Improving Mothers' Care. Lessons learned to inform maternity care from the UK and Ireland. Confidential enquiries into maternal deaths and morbidity 2014–16.* Oxford: MBRRACE/NPEU. Available from: https://www.npeu.ox.ac.uk/mbrrace-uk/reports. [Accessed 12 April 2019].

Moran, P., & Findley, M. (2013). Addictive disorders. In E. Robson, & J. Waugh (Eds.), *Medical disorders in pregnancy: A manual for midwives* (2nd ed.) (pp. 299–318). Chichester, WSussex: Wiley Blackwell.

Moran, P. (2017). Substance misuse in pregnancy. In D. James, P. Steer, C. Weiner, B. Gonik, & S. Robson (Eds.), *High risk pregnancy: Management options* (5th ed.) (pp. 779–807). Cambridge: Cambridge University Press.

National Institute of Health and Care Excellence (NICE). (2010). *CG110.* Pregnancy and complex social factors: A model for service provision for pregnant women with complex social factors [online]. Last updated August 2018. London: NICE. Available from: https://www.nice.org.uk/guidance/cg110. [Accessed 14 April 2019].

National Institute of Health and Care Excellence (NICE). (2014). CG192. Antenatal and postnatal mental health: Clinical management and service guidance [online]. Last updated April 2018. London: NICE. Available from: https://www.nice.org.uk/guidance/cg192. [Accessed 4 April 2019].

National Institute for Health and Clinical Excellence (NICE). (2019). *Valproate in children, young people and adults: Summary of NICE guidance and safety advice* [online]. Available from: https://www.nice.org.uk/guidance/cg137/resources/valproate-in-children-young-people-and-adults-summary-of-nice-guidance-and-safety-advice-pdf-6723784045. [Accessed 22 June 2019].

Nursing and Midwifery Council (NMC), 2019. *Standards of proficiency for midwives.* London: NMC. Available from: https://www.nmc.org.uk/globalassets/sitedocuments/standards/standards-of-proficiency-for-midwives.pdf . [Accessed 20 November 2019].

Price, S. (Ed.). (2007). *Mental health in pregnancy and childbirth.* Edinburgh: Churchill Livingstone/Elsevier.

Prothiaden 75mg tablets. Teofarma. Last updated on the BNF [online] April 2019.

SmPC from the eMC. Cyclogest 200mg and 400mg pessaries. LD Collins & Co Ltd. Last updated on the eMC 28/09/2018.

SmPC from the eMC. Fluoxetine 20mg capsules. Accord Healthcare Ltd. Last updated on the eMC 09/03/2017.

SmPC from the eMC. Methadone 1mg/mL oral solution. Martindale Pharma. Last updated on the eMC 31/03/2017.

SmPC from the eMC. Pridel® 200mg and 400 mg tablets. SANOFI. Last updated on the eMC 20/09/2018.

SmPC from the eMC. Pridel® 520 mg/5 mL oral liquid. SANOFI. Last updated on the eMC 20/09/2018.

SmPC from the eMC. Prozac® 20mg capsules and Prozac® 20mg/5mL oral solution. Eli Lilly and company Ltd. Last updated on the eMC 14/05/2018.

Weiner, C., & Mason, C. (2017). Medication. In D. James, P. Steer, C. Weiner, B. Gonik, & S. Robson (Eds.), *High risk pregnancy: Management options* (5th ed.) (pp. 808–846). Cambridge: Cambridge University Press.

Antiemetics

These are drugs used to prevent or lessen nausea and vomiting. Some of these preparations may also be antipsychotics or antihistamines.

The student should be aware of:

- the actions of analgesics on the cerebral cortex
- the results of administration of the antipsychotic antiemetics, i.e. their potentiating effects
- the appropriateness of treatment using antiemetics, especially in early pregnancy.

BP
Prochlorperazine maleate or mesilate

Proprietary
Prochlorperazine (Accord-UK Ltd)
Prochlorperazine injection (ADVANZ Pharma)
Stemetil (SANOFI)
Prochlorperazine (non-proprietary, see BNF for details)

Group
Antiemetic – antipsychotic

Uses/indications
Prophylaxis with the use of opioid analgesic, or with excessive emesis

Type of drug
POM, Midwives' Exemptions

Presentation
Ampoules, tablets

Dosage
IM: 12.5 mg 6–8 hourly (eMC 9/4/2019)
Oral: initially 20 mg then 10 mg after 2 hours
Prevention of emesis: 5–10 mg b.d. or t.d.s. (eMC
29/5/2019) Migraine or labyrinthitis: 5 mg t.d.s.
Route of admin
IM, oral, P.R.
Contraindications
Pregnancy, myasthenia gravis, cardiovascular and
respiratory disease, epilepsy, phaeochromocytoma,
liver or renal dysfunction, hypothyroidism
Side effects
*Can cause prolonged labour and should be withheld
until 3–4 cm dilution,* drowsiness, pallor, hypother-
mia, extrapyramidal effects, postural hypotension with
tachycardia, liver dysfunction
Interactions
Alcohol – increases the sedative effect, particularly
respiratory depression
Antacids – interfere with the absorption of oral Stemetil
Anaesthetics – increases their hypertensive effect
Antiepileptics – phenobarbital – decreases plasma concentrations but is not thought to be clinically significant
Antihistamines – increased risk of ventricular arrhythmias with terfenadine
Antihypertensives – with methyldopa there is an
increased risk of extrapyramidal effects
Pharmacodynamic properties
A potent phenothiazine neuroleptic used in nausea
and vomiting, and in schizophrenia, acute mania and
the management of anxiety
Fetal risk
In the first trimester there are reports of congenital
defects associated with repeated use even at low
doses, but single or occasional low doses appear safe;
extrapyramidal symptoms in the neonate, lethargy and
tremor, low Apgar Score, paradoxical hyperexcitability

Breastfeeding
Amount probably too small to be excreted but avoid
unless absolutely necessary; the manufacturer recommends against therapy during breastfeeding

BP
Metoclopramide hydrochloride

Proprietary
Maxolon® (ADVANZ Pharma)
Metoclopramide hydrochloride (non-proprietary, see
BNF for details)

Group
Antiemetic

Uses/indications
Nausea, vomiting
30 mg daily in divided doses

Type of drug
POM

Presentation
Tablets, ampoules, infusion, oral suspension

Dosage
10 mg as single dose, repeated up to three times per
day, max 30 mg per day (eMC 27/2/2019 n b/3/2019)

Route of admin
IM, oral, continuous infusion or slow IV

Contraindications
Hepatic and renal impairment; may cause hypertension in phaeochromocytoma; caution in epilepsy

Side effects
Extrapyramidal effects, hyperprolactinaemia

Interactions
Analgesics – increases the absorption of aspirin and paracetamol, thereby enhancing their effect
Opioid analgesics – antagonize the effect on gastrointestinal activity
SSRIs – use with care

Pharmacodynamic properties
Action of metoclopramide is closely associated with the parasympathetic nervous control of the upper GI tract. It encourages normal peristaltic action and is indicated in conditions where disturbed GI motility is an underlying factor

Fetal risk
Use with caution specifically in first trimester; there is no information on the long-term evaluation of infants exposed in utero

Breastfeeding
Use with caution as there is a theoretical risk of potent CNS effects

---

BP
Cyclizine hydrochloride or lactate

Proprietary
Cyclizine (Valoid) (ADVANZ Pharma)
Cyclizine hydrochloride (non-proprietary, see BNF for details),

Group
Anticholinergic – antiemetic

Uses/indications
Prevention and treatment of nausea and vomiting

Continued

Type of drug
POM, Midwives' Exemptions

Presentation
Tablets, ampoules

Dosage
Oral: 50 mg, max three doses per day (eMC 16/10/2018)
IM or IV: 50 mg can be given t.d.s.
Post-op: slow IV injection 20 min before the end of surgery (eMC 6/8/2018)

Route of admin
Oral, IM, IV

Contraindications
Hypersensitivity to cyclizine, cardiac disease

Side effects
Hypotension, fall in cardiac output, urticaria, rash, drowsiness, oropharyngeal dryness, tachycardia, blurred vision, urinary retention, constipation

Interactions
Alcohol – enhances the effect of cyclizine
Analgesics – enhances soporific effect of pethidine
Anticholinergics – concomitant use gives enhanced effects
CNS suppressants – enhances the effect of cyclizine

Pharmacodynamic properties
A histamine H_1-receptor antagonist, cyclizine has a low incidence of drowsiness but has antiemetic and anticholinergic properties. The exact mechanism is unknown, but it is thought to act to increase lower oesophageal sphincter tone, and it may also have an inhibitory effect on the emetic centre located in the midbrain

Fetal risk
Manufacturer advises that animal studies indicate teratogenicity

Breastfeeding
No data available from controlled studies in breast-feeding women, but considered moderately safe

References and Recommended Reading

Berlin, C. (2013). Medications and the breastfeeding mother. In D. Mattison (Ed.), *Clinical pharmacology during pregnancy* (pp. 41–54). Edinburgh: Elsevier.

Briggs, G., Freeman, R., Towers, C., & Forinash, A. (2017). *Drugs in pregnancy and lactation: A reference guide to fetal and neonatal risk* (11th ed.). Philadelphia: Wolters Kluwer.

Doughty, R., & Waugh, J. (2013). Metabolic disorders. In E. Robson, & J. Waugh (Eds.), *Medical disorders in pregnancy: A manual for midwives* (2nd ed.) (pp. 241–254). Chichester, WSussex: Wiley Blackwell.

Herbert, M. (2013). Impact of pregnancy on maternal pharmacokinetics of medications. In D. Mattison (Ed.), *Clinical pharmacology during pregnancy* (pp. 17–40) Edinburgh: Elsevier.

Jordan, S. (2010). Antiemetics. In S. Jordan (Ed.), *Pharmacology for midwives: The evidence base for safe practice* (2nd ed.) (pp. 121–142). Basingstoke: Palgrave.

Jordan, S., & MacDonald, S. (2017). Pharmacology and the midwife. In S. MacDonald, & C Johnson (Eds.), *Mayes' midwifery, A text book for midwives* (15th ed.) (pp. 158–174). Edinburgh: Elsevier.

Nursing and Midwifery Council (NMC), 2019. *Standards of proficiency for midwives.* London: NMC. Available from: https://www.nmc.org.uk/globalassets/sitedocuments/standards/standards-of-proficiency-for-midwives.pdf. [Accessed 20 November 2019].

Rankin, J. (2017). Fluid, electrolyte and acid-base balance. In J. Rankin (Ed.), *Physiology in childbearing with anatomy and related biosciences* (pp. 207–216). Edinburgh: Elsevier.

Royal College of Obstetricians and Gynaecologists (RCOG). (2016). *CTG69 The management of nausea and vomiting of pregnancy and hyperemesis gravidarum.* Available from: https://www.rcog.org.uk/globalassets/documents/guidelines/green-top-guidelines/gtg69-hyperemesis.pdf. [Accessed 10 June 2019].

SmPC from the eMC. Cyclizine 50mg tablets (Valoid®). ADVANZ Pharma. Last updated on the eMC 16/10/2018.

SmPC from the eMC. Cyclizine lactate 50 mg/mL injection. ADVANZ Pharma. Last updated on the eMC 6/8/2018.

SmPC from the eMC. Maxolon 10mg tablets. ADVANZ Pharma. Last updated on the eMC 27/2/2019.

SmPC from the eMC. Maxolon hydrochloride 5mg/mL injection. ADVANZ Pharma. Last updated on the eMC 4/3/2019.

SmPC from the eMC. Prochlorperazine 5mg tablets. Accord-UK Ltd. Last updated on the eMC 29/5/2019.

SmPC from the eMC. Prochlorperazine (prochlorperazine mesilate) 12.5mg/mL, as 1mL & 2mL injection. ADVANZ Pharma. Last updated on the eMC 9/4/2019.

SmPC from the eMC. Stemetil® 5mg tablets. SANOFI. Last updated on the eMC 21/3/2019.

SmPC from the eMC. Stemetil® injection. SANOFI. Last updated on the eMC 22/3/2019.

SmPC from the eMC. Stemetil®syrup. SANOFI. Last updated on the eMC 21/3/2019.

Weiner, C., & Mason, C. (2017). Medication. In D. James, P. Steer, C. Weiner, B. Gonik, & S. Robson (Eds.), *High risk pregnancy: Management options* (5th ed.) (pp. 808–846). Cambridge: Cambridge University Press.

van der Woude, C., Kanis, S., & De Lima, A. (2017). Gastrointestinal and liver diseases in pregnancy. In D. James, P. Steer, C. Weiner, B. Gonik, & S. Robson (Eds.), *High risk pregnancy: Management options* (5th ed.) (pp. 1236–1272). Cambridge: Cambridge University Press.

9

Antifungals

These are drugs used to combat fungal infections. They can be ingested or applied topically, depending on the infection.

The student should be aware of:

- common fungal infections in pregnancy and postnatal care
- the physiology and pathophysiology that allow these infections to flourish
- the appropriateness of the antifungal treatment prescribed.

BP
Nystatin

Proprietary
Nystan® suspension (Sandoz Ltd)
Nystaform® cream (Typharm Ltd)
Nystatin (non-proprietary, see BNF for details)

Group
Antifungal

Uses/indications
Candidiasis in the mouth, oesophagus or intestinal tract

Type of drug
POM, Midwives' Exemptions

Presentation
Oral suspension (yellow), cream (light yellow)

Continued

Dosage
Adult: Oral – 500 000 units q.d.s. for 7 days, i.e. 5 mL suspension (contains sugar) (eMC 15/3/2017); cream – 100 000 units/g 2–3 times per day to affected skin (eMC 12/1/2018)
Paediatric: Oral – 100 000 units q.d.s. for 7 days, i.e. 1 mL suspension (contains sugar) (eMC 15/3/2017)

Route of admin
Oral, topical

Contraindications
Hypersensitivity to constituents

Side effects
Nausea, vomiting, hypersensitivity

Interactions
No data available

Pharmacodynamic properties
Antifungal that is not absorbed by the gastrointestinal tract, skin or vagina, and that inhibits growth of microbes, mostly yeasts and yeast-like fungi, e.g. *Candida albicans*

Fetal risk
No reports of complications after administration in pregnancy

Breastfeeding
Not known to be secreted in breast milk; manufacturers recommend caution

---

BP
Clotrimazole

Proprietary
Canesten® vaginal cream or pessary (Bayer plc)
Canesten® Oral Capsule (Fluconazole 150 mg) (Bayer plc)
Diflucan™ Oral Capsule (Pfizer Limited)
Clotrimazole (non-proprietary, see BNF for details)

Group
Antifungal

Uses/indications
Candidiasis

Type of drug
POM, GSL, Pharmacy only (oral)

Presentation
Cream (topical – internal and external), pessaries (vaginal), capsule

Dosage
See manufacturers' instructions

Route of admin
P.V. during pregnancy the pessary should be inserted without using an applicator, and topically to the external vulval area. Oral – not recommended during pregnancy or breastfeeding – see manufacturers' information

Contraindications
Hypersensitivity

Side effects
Occasional local irritation

Interactions
Antifungals – may reduce the efficacy of other drugs used in fungal disease, e.g. nystatin
Contraceptives – may affect latex condoms and diaphragms

Pharmacodynamic properties
Broad-spectrum antifungal effective against proliferating fungi, e.g. yeast, mould, dermatophytes, and others. The antimycotic effect against the cell wall releases hydrogen peroxide and causes cell death

Fetal risk
No adverse effects; no epidemiological data available, despite use over time

Breastfeeding
Considered safe as minimal absorption

References and Recommended Reading

Berlin, C. (2013). Medications and the breastfeeding mother. In D. Mattison (Ed.), *Clinical Pharmacology During Pregnancy* (pp. 41–54). Edinburgh: Elsevier.

Briggs, G., Freeman, R., Towers, C., & Forinash, A. (2017). *Drugs in Pregnancy and Lactation: A reference guide to fetal and neonatal risk* (11th ed.). Philadelphia: Wolters Kluwer.

Herbert, M. (2013). Impact of pregnancy on maternal pharmacokinetics of medications. In D. Mattison (Ed.), *Clinical Pharmacology During Pregnancy* (pp. 17–40). Edinburgh: Elsevier.

Johnson, R., & Taylor, W. (2016). *Skills for Midwifery Practice* (4th ed.). Edinburgh: Elsevier.

Nursing and Midwifery Council (NMC). (2019). *Standards of proficiency for midwives*. London: NMC. Available from: https://www.nmc.org.uk/globalassets/sitedocuments/standards/standards-of-proficiency-for-midwives.pdf. [Accessed 20 April 2019].

SmPC from the eMC. Canesten® 2% vaginal cream. Bayer plc. Last updated on the eMC 16/1/2018.

SmPC from the eMC. Canesten® 10% vaginal cream. Bayer plc. Last updated on the eMC 12/1/2018.

SmPC from the eMC. Canesten® 100mg pessary. Bayer plc. Last updated on the eMC 16/1/2018.

SmPC from the eMC. Canesten® 150mg capsule. Bayer plc. Last updated on the eMC 3/10/2018.

SmPC from the eMC. Diflucan™ 150mg capsule. Pfizer Limited. Last updated on the eMC 22/3/2019.

SmPC from the eMC. Nystatin® 100,000 iu/mL oral suspension. Sandoz Limited. Last updated on the eMC 15/3/2017.

SmPC from the eMC. Nystatin/Chlorhexidine hydrochloride 100,000 iu/g /1% cream. Typharm Limited. Last updated on the eMC 15/6/2017.

Tait, M. (2010). Antimicrobial agents. In S. Jordan (Ed.), *Pharmacology for Midwives: The Evidence Base for Safe Practice* (2nd ed.) (pp. 303–326). Basingstoke: Palgrave Macmillan.

Weiner, C., & Mason, C. (2017). Medication. In D. James, P. Steer, C. Weiner, B. Gonik, & S. Robson (Eds.), *High Risk Pregnancy: Management Options* (5th ed.) (pp. 808–846). Cambridge: Cambridge University Press.

Further Reading

Breastfeeding network. (2017). *Thrush and Breastfeeding factsheet*. Available from: https://www.breastfeedingnetwork.org.uk/thrush-detailed/. [Accessed 21 October 2019].

National Institute for Health and Care Excellence (NICE). (2017). *Clinical Knowledge Summary: Candidias – female genital*. Available from https://cks.nice.org.uk/candida-female-genital. [Accessed 4 July 2019]. https://cks.nice.org.uk/candida-female-genital#!scenario:4. See specifically scenario 4.

National Institute for Health and Care Excellence (NICE). (2017). *Clinical Knowledge Summary: Candidias – oral*. Available from: https://cks.nice.org.uk/candida-oral. [Accessed 4 July 2019]. https://cks.nice.org.uk/candida-oral#!scenario. See specifically scenario 1.

10

Antihistamines

The term 'antihistamine' refers to H_2 receptor antagonists and are subdivided into sedating antihistamines and non-sedating antihistamines. Uses include:

- antiemetics for nausea and vomiting (see Chapter 8)
- emergency treatment (anaphylactic shock) (see Chapter 15)
- allergy relief
- cholestasis of pregnancy
- premedication and sedation
- insomnia
- relief of colds and coughs.

Histamine is present in animal tissues and some release occurs after injury, but also after an allergic reaction, and gives rise to urticaria, asthma, hay fever and ultimately anaphylaxis. Antihistamines are palliative agents because they neither destroy nor prevent the release of histamine, but act by blocking access to histamine receptor sites and thereby inhibiting an allergic reaction. Antihistamines are usually thought of as being taken orally, but they can be injected; for example, chlorpheniramine and promethazine are used as adjuncts to adrenaline (epinephrine) in the treatment of anaphylaxis (see Chapter 15). They can also be used intranasally, intraocularly and topically.

The student should be aware of:

- the physiology related to allergic response
- the most common factors causing allergic response

- recognition of and treatment for anaphylactic shock
- interactions of drug therapy that may produce an allergic response.

Midwives can administer 'adrenaline 1:1000' for anaphylaxis under the Midwives' Exemptions (The Human Medicines Regulations 2012, Schedule 17, Part 3, section 2).

BP
Chlorpheniramine maleate

Proprietary
Piriton (GlaxoSmithKline Consumer Healthcare)
Chlorpheniramine maleate injection (Wockhardt UK Ltd)
Chlorpheniramine maleate (non-proprietary, see BNF for details)

Group
Antihistamine – sedative

Uses/indications
Symptomatic control of all allergic conditions responsive to antihistamines, including hay fever, vasomotor rhinitis, urticaria, angioneurotic oedema, food allergy, drug and serum reactions, insect bites. Symptomatic relief of itch associated with chickenpox. **Anaphylaxis** – see Chapter 15

Type of drug
POM, GSL

Presentation
Tablets (4 mg), syrup (2 mg/5 mL), ampoules (10 mg/mL)

Dosage
General use: Oral 4 mg 4–6 hourly to a max 24 mg daily IM (eMC 17/10/2016) or IV over 1 min, 10 mg, repeated if required up to max 4 doses in 24 hours (eMC 10/11 2017)
Emergency use: see Chapter 15

Route of admin

Oral, IM, IV (see Chapter 15 on emergency drugs)

Contraindications

Epilepsy, hepatic disease, asthma, patients who are hypersensitive to antihistamines or to any of the tablet ingredients, and patients who have been treated with MAOIs within the last 14 days

Side effects

Drowsiness, lassitude, dizziness, dry mouth, blurred vision, headache, gastrointestinal disturbances; IV may cause transient hypotension, CNS stimulation and may be an irritant; inability to concentrate, hepatitis – including jaundice, urinary retention, palpitations, arrhythmias, hypotension, chest tightness, blood disorders including haemolytic anaemia

Allergic reactions: exfoliative dermatitis, photosensitivity, twitching, urticaria, muscle weakness, incoordination, tinnitus, depression, irritability, nightmares

Interactions

Alcohol – potentiates sedative action

Antidepressants – enhance sedative effect – anticholinergic effect intensified with MAOIs

Antidiabetics – depressed thrombocyte count

Antiepileptics – inhibits metabolism of phenytoin

Antihistamines – concomitant therapy NOT recommended

Anxiolytics and hypnotics – enhance the sedative effect

Pharmacodynamic properties

Chlorpheniramine is a potent antihistamine (H_1 antagonist) that diminishes or abolishes the actions of histamine in the body by competitive reversible blockade of histamine H_1-receptor sites on tissues. Chlorpheniramine also has anticholinergic activity preventing the release of histamine, prostaglandins and leukotrienes, and the migration of inflammatory mediators. The actions of chlorpheniramine include inhibition of histamine on smooth muscle, capillary permeability and hence reduction of oedema and raised, red, itchy areas of skin in hypersensitivity reactions such as allergy and anaphylaxis

Fetal risk

No adequate data available in relation to chlorpheniramine maleate in pregnant women. Use during the third trimester may result in reactions in the newborn or premature neonates. Not to be used during pregnancy unless considered essential by a physician

Breastfeeding

Chlorpheniramine maleate and other antihistamines may inhibit lactation and may be secreted in breast milk. Manufacturers recommend not to be used during lactation

Other antihistamines that are used in the relief of allergies, including hay fever, are:

Older antihistamines: Alimemazine tartrate, Hydroxyzine which may cause sedation, although Chlorphenamine and Cyclizine are less sedating.

Non-sedating antihistamines: Acrivastine, Bilastine, Cetirizine, Desloratidine, Fexofenadine, Levocertirizine, Loratadine, and Mizolastine (Source: BNF, last accessed 10 June 2019).

ALL are not recommended for use in pregnancy, and the risk of embryotoxicity is significantly high with loratadine and fexofenadine.

References and Recommended Reading

Berlin, C. (2013). Medications and the breastfeeding mother. In D. Mattison (Ed.), *Clinical Pharmacology During Pregnancy* (pp. 41–54). Edinburgh: Elsevier.

Briggs, G., Freeman, R., Towers, C., & Forinash, A. (2017). *Drugs in Pregnancy and Lactation: A reference guide to fetal and neonatal risk* (11th ed.). Philadelphia: Wolters Kluwer.

Herbert, M. (2013). Impact of pregnancy on maternal pharmacokinetics of medications. In D. Mattison (Ed.), *Clinical Pharmacology During Pregnancy* (pp. 17–40). Edinburgh: Elsevier.

Her Majesty's Stationary Office. (2012). *The Human Medicines Regulations 2012*. London: HMSO. Available from: http://www.legislation.gov.uk/uksi/2012/1916/pdfs/uksi_20121916_en.pdf. [Accessed 12 April 2019].

Her Majesty's Stationary Office. (2014). *The Human Medicines (Amendment) Regulations 2014*. London: HMSO. Available from: http://www.legislation.gov.uk/uksi/2014/490/pdfs/uksi_20140490_en.pdf. [Accessed 12 April 2019].

Her Majesty's Stationary Office. (2016). *The Human Medicines (Amendment) Regulations 2016*. London: HMSO. Available from: https://www.legislation.gov.uk/uksi/2016/186/pdfs/uksi_20160186_en.pdf. [Accessed 16 April 2019].

Jordan, S. (2010). Anti-emetics. In S. Jordan (Ed.), *Pharmacology for midwives: The evidence base for safe practice* (2nd ed.) (pp. 121–142). Basingstoke: Palgrave. See 134-139 specifically.

Jordan, S., & MacDonald, S. (2017). Pharmacology and the midwife. In S. MacDonald, & G. Johnson (Eds.), *Mayes' Midwifery: A Text Book for Midwives* (15th ed.) (pp. 158–174). Edinburgh: Elsevier.

Nursing and Midwifery Council (NMC). (2015). *update 2018. The Code - Professional standards of practice and behaviour for nurses, midwives and nursing associates*. London: NMC.

Nursing and Midwifery Council (NMC). (2017). *updated 2019. Practicing as a Midwife in the UK*. London: NMC.

Nursing and Midwifery Council (NMC). (2019). *Standards of proficiency for midwives*. London: NMC. Available from: https://www.nmc.org.uk/globalassets/sitedocuments/standards/standards-of-proficiency-for-midwives.pdf. [Accessed 20 April 2019].

SmPC from the eMC. Chlorphenamine maleate 10mg/mL solution for injection. Wockhardt UK Ltd. Last updated on the eMC 10/11/2017.

SmPC from the eMC. Piriton® tablets. GlaxoSmithKline Consumer Healthcare. Last updated on the eMC 27/10/2016.

SmPC from the eMC. Piriton® syrup. GlaxoSmithKline Consumer Healthcare. Last updated on the eMC 27/10/2016.

Weiner, C., & Mason, C. (2017). Medication. In D. James, P. Steer, C. Weiner, B. Gonik, & S. Robson (Eds.), *High Risk Pregnancy: Management Options* (5th ed.) (pp. 808–846). Cambridge: Cambridge University Press.

11

Antihypertensives

These are substances used to control or modify blood pressure, either by reducing peripheral resistance or blocking α or β adrenoreceptors in the heart, or by reducing the central flow of impulses to the sympathetic nerves and decreasing the release of noradrenaline (norepinephrine) at adrenergic nerve endings.

The student should be aware of:

- the physiology and pathophysiology of blood pressure
- the aetiology, pathophysiology and progression of pregnancy-induced hypertension and pre-eclampsia
- the difference between chronic hypertension (mild, moderate or severe), gestational hypertension, pre-eclampsia, severe pre-eclampsia and eclampsia (NICE 2010, p. 5)
- the maternal and fetal sequelae of therapy using these substances
- the local protocols for treatment in cases of eclampsia (see Chapter 15, Emergency drugs, e.g. magnesium sulfate).

NOTE: NICE guideline (CG 107, 2010, p. 18 & p. 20) lists other medications that may be used during childbearing in some instances: ***atenolol, captopril, enalapril*** and ***metoprolol***. Specific information for these medications should be sought if used for treatments in local NHS Trusts.

BP
Nifedipine

Proprietary
Adipine MR (Chesni Ltd)
Adalat LA (Bayer PLC)
Nifedipine (non-proprietary, see BNF for details)

Group
Calcium channel blocker, hypotensive, vasodilator

Uses/indications
Hypertensive crisis, uncontrolled hypertension. Myometrial relaxant – see Chapter 20

Type of drug
POM

Presentation
(Soft) capsules, tablets (modified or prolonged release)

Dosage
Hypertension: 20 mg stat, 20–80 mg daily in divided doses 12 hours apart (eMC 12/10/2017)
Tocolytic: see Chapter 20 for regimen if used as myometrial relaxant

Route of admin
Oral

Contraindications
Continuous use in pregnancy, breastfeeding, hypersensitivity

Side effects
Headache, flushing, dizziness, oedema, may inhibit labour
CAUTION: stop treatment if ischaemic pain occurs within 30–60 min of administration; treatment with short-acting nifedipine, i.e. during a crisis, can induce an exaggerated fall in blood pressure and reflex tachycardia, which may cause complications such as cerebrovascular accident/ischaemia or myocardial ischaemia
EXTREME CAUTION when using magnesium sulfate

Interactions

Do not take with grapefruit juice

Antihypertensives – causes severe hypotension and possible heart failure

Cimetidine – potentiates the hypotensive effect as metabolism of nifedipine is inhibited Phenytoin – concomitant administration can reduce the effect of nifedipine – monitor plasma levels of anticonvulsants

Erythromycin – may potentiate nifedipine effects

Insulin – possible impaired glucose tolerance

Pharmacodynamic properties

Selective calcium channel blocker with mostly vascular effects. It is a specific and potent calcium antagonist that relaxes smooth arterial muscle, causing arteries to widen, thereby reducing the resistance in coronary and peripheral circulation. This reduces blood pressure and decreases the heart's overall workload

Fetal risk

Contraindicated in pregnancy before week 20; toxicity and teratogenicity in animals; hypotensive effect can reduce placental flow and cause decrease in fetal oxygenation; may inhibit labour

Breastfeeding

Excreted in breast milk; therefore manufacturers advise avoidance

BP

Methyldopa

Proprietary

Aldomet (Aspen)

Methyldopa BP (Intrapharm Laboratories Ltd)

Methyldopa (non-proprietary, see BNF for details)

Group

Centrally acting antihypertensive

Continued 131

Uses/indications
Hypertension in pregnancy, hypertensive crisis where immediate effect is not necessary, can be used by asthmatics

Type of drug
POM

Presentation
Tablets

Dosage
Oral: 250 mg b.d. (or t.d.s.) max 3 g/day, gradually increased at intervals of 2 days or more (eMC 3/9/2016)

Route of admin
Oral

Contraindications
History of depression, liver disease, phaeochromocytoma, concurrent treatment with MAOIs, porphyria, history of hepatic or renal dysfunction

Side effects
Reduced if under 1 g/day, dry mouth, sedation, depression, fluid retention, haemolytic anaemia, SLE-like syndrome, postural hypotension, gastrointestinal disturbances, dizziness, headache, numbness, hyperprolactinaemia, nightmares, mild psychosis, blood disorders, nasal congestion, nerve and joint pain, hepatic disorders; may interfere with laboratory results – 20% have a positive DCT – advise laboratory of treatment if requiring crossmatch

Interactions
Sympathomimetics, phenothiazines, tricyclic antidepressants and MAOIs – diminish effect
Alcohol – enhances hypotensive effect
Anaesthetics – enhances hypotensive effect ++
Analgesics – NSAIDs enhance hypotensive effect
Antihypertensives – potentiate hypotensive effect
Anxiolytics and hypnotics – enhance hypotensive effect
Corticosteroids – antagonize hypotensive effect
Contraceptives – antagonize hypotensive effect
Iron – possible reduction in the bioavailability of ferrous sulphate or ferrous gluconate if ingested with methyldopa
Salbutamol – use with caution as it can potentiate the hypotensive effect

Pharmacodynamic properties
Methyldopa is metabolized to α-methylnoradrenaline, which lowers arterial pressure (stimulates central inhibitory α-adrenergic receptors), limiting neurotransmission, and/or reduction of plasma renin activity. Withdrawal of the drug is followed by a return of hypertension within 48 hours

Fetal risk
Crosses the placental barrier and is present in cord blood; there are theoretical risks of toxicity/teratogenicity including neural development (IQ and links to ADHD)

Breastfeeding
Found in breast milk, and although there are no obvious effects the manufacturer advises that lactating mothers be warned of its presence and possible risk, but does not advise avoidance

BP
Hydralazine hydrochloride

Proprietary
Apresoline (ADVANZ Pharma)
Hydralazine hydrochloride (non-proprietary, see BNF for details)

Group
Antihypertensive – vasodilator

Uses/indications
Raised diastolic blood pressure used concomitantly with other therapies, e.g. β-blockers or during a hypertensive crisis

Type of drug
POM

Presentation
Tablets, injection, powder for reconstitution

Dosage
Oral: 25–50 mg b.d.
Slow IV injection: 5–10 mg over 20 min, repeated after 20–30 min – diluted with sodium chloride 0.9%
IV infusion: 200–300 mcg/min
Maintenance: 5–150 mcg/min (eMC 3/1/2019)

Route of admin
Oral, IV injection or infusion

Contraindications
SLE, tachycardia, hepatic, renal or cardiac dysfunction, or cerebrovascular accident

Side effects
Nausea, postural hypotension, tachycardia, palpitations, flushing, fluid retention, after prolonged or high-dose therapy SLE-like syndrome, headache, dizziness, joint, muscle and nerve pain, nasal congestion, blood disorders, liver and renal disorders

Interactions

Alcohol – enhances hypotensive effect

Anaesthetics – enhance hypotensive effect

Analgesics – NSAIDs enhance hypotensive effect

Antihypertensives – enhance hypotensive effect

Anxiolytics and hypnotics – enhance the hypotensive effects

Contraceptives – combined oral contraceptives antagonize the hypotensive effect

Pharmacodynamic properties

Acts on the smooth muscle tissue surrounding the arteries, causing them to relax and hence the blood pressure to fall

Fetal risk

Toxicity in animals, therefore considered a teratogen, although there are no reported links to congenital defects in humans. Avoid before the third trimester, but there are no reports of serious harm

Breastfeeding

Passes into breast milk, but no known adverse side effects thus considered safe, but infant requires monitoring

BP

Labetalol hydrochloride

Proprietary

Trandate (RPH Pharmaceuticals AB)

Labetalol (non-proprietary, see BNF for details)

Group

Antihypertensive – α and β adrenoreceptor blocker

Uses/indications

Hypertension in pregnancy, hypertensive crisis

Type of drug

POM

Continued 135

Presentation
Tablets, ampoules

Dosage
Oral: initial dose 100 mg b.d. increased at weekly intervals by 100 mg b.d., to 200 mg b.d. In the second and third trimesters further dose titration to t.d.s., ranging from 100 to 400 mg t.d.s.; can be increased up to 800 mg in three to four evenly divided doses/day (max 2.4 g daily) (eMC 25/5/2017)
IV injection: 50 mg over 1 min repeated after 5 min (max 200 mg)
IV infusion: 20 mg/hour doubled after 30 min (max 160 mg/hour) (eMC 22/3/2019)

Route of admin
Oral, IV injection or infusion

Contraindications
Asthma, chronic obstructive airway disease, wheezing, phaeochromocytoma, bradycardia, sensitivity to labetalol, heart block, Raynaud's disease, use with caution in patients with psoriasis

Side effects
Postural hypotension – particularly 3 hours after IV administration, tiredness, weakness, epigastric pain, difficulty with micturition, scalp tingling, tremor in pregnant patients

Interactions

Alcohol – enhances hypotensives effect as delays metabolism of labetalol

Anaesthetics – enhance hypotensive effect

Analgesics – NSAIDs enhance hypotensive effects

Antacids – cimetidine inhibits the metabolism and therefore increases the plasma concentration of labetalol

Antidepressants – tricyclics cause tremor; MAOIs not recommended

Antidiabetics – enhanced hypoglycaemic effects and masks warning signs such as tremor Antihistamines – increased risk of ventricular arrhythmia with terfenadine

Antihypertensives – concomitant use may cause severe hypotension

Anxiolytics and hypnotics - enhance the hypotensive effect

Corticosteroids – antagonize the hypotensive effect

Ergometrine – increases peripheral vasoconstriction

Contraceptives – combined oral contraceptives antagonize the hypotensive effect

Pharmacodynamic properties

Works by blocking peripheral arteriolar α receptors and this reduces peripheral resistance. A concurrent β-blockade protects the heart from any reflux effects. Cardiac output is not significantly reduced at rest or after moderate exercise, i.e. the increase in systolic pressure during exercise is reduced and the diastolic pressure remains essentially normal

Continued

Fetal risk

Manufacturers advise labetalol should be used only in the first trimester if benefit outweighs risk; caution in use – β-blockers reduce placental perfusion, leading to a risk of intrauterine death, premature delivery, fetal growth deficiency, and increased risk of neonatal hypoglycaemia and bradycardia, respiratory depression and neonatal jaundice. The risk is greater in severe hypertension and with multiple therapy, although these effects may be due to the disease itself and not the therapy. These symptoms can develop 1–2 days after delivery

Breastfeeding

Excreted in breast milk; although manufacturers recommend avoidance, no known adverse side effects (NICE 2010)

References and Recommended Reading

Berlin, C. (2013). Medications and the breastfeeding mother. In D. Mattison (Ed.), *Clinical Pharmacology During Pregnancy* (pp. 41–54). Edinburgh: Elsevier.

Briggs, G., Freeman, R., Towers, C., & Forinash, A. (2017). *Drugs in Pregnancy and Lactation: A reference guide to fetal and neonatal risk* (11th ed.). Philadelphia: Wolters Kluwer.

Gilbert, E. (2011). *Hypertensive disorders. Manual of High Risk Pregnancy and Delivery* (5th ed.). St Louis: Mosby/Elsevier, 416–459.

Jordan, S. (2010). Cardiovascular disorders in pregnancy. In S. Jordan (Ed.), *Pharmacology for Midwives: The Evidence Base for Safe Practice* (2nd ed.) (pp. 223–255). Basingstoke: Palgrave Macmillan.

Jordan, S., & MacDonald, S. (2017). Pharmacology and the midwife. In S. MacDonald, & G. Johnson (Eds.), *Mayes' Midwifery: A Text Book for Midwives* (15th ed.) (pp. 158–174). Edinburgh: Elsevier.

McEwan, T. (2017). Cardiac and hypertensive disorders. In J. Rankin, J (Ed.), *Physiology in childbearing with anatomy and related biosciences* (pp. 335–341). Edinburgh: Elsevier.

National Institute of Health and Care Excellence (NICE). (2010). *CG107. Hypertension in pregnancy: Diagnosis and management* [online]. Last updated January 2011. London: NICE. Available from: https://www.nice.org.uk/guidance/cg107. [Accessed 4 April 2019]. Latest NICE pathway (June 2017) available from: http://pathways.nice.org.uk/pathways/hypertension-in-pregnancy. [Accessed 10 June 2019].

Nursing and Midwifery Council (NMC). (2019). *Standards of proficiency for midwives*. London: NMC. Available from: https://www.nmc.org.uk/globalassets/sitedocuments/standards/standards-of-proficiency-for-midwives.pdf. [Accessed 20 April 2019].

SmPC from the eMC. Adalat® 20mg tablets. Bayer plc. Last updated on the eMC 12/10/2017.

SmPC from the eMC. Adipine 10mg tablets. Chiesi Limited. Last updated on the eMC 16/9/2016.

SmPC from the eMC. Aldomet® 250mg tablets. Aspen. Last updated on the eMC 30/9/2016.

SmPC from the eMC. Hydralazine 20mg powder for solution for injection/infusion. ADVANZ Pharma. Last updated on the eMC 3/1/2019.

SmPC from the eMC. Labetalol hydrochloride 5mg/mL solution for injection. RPH Pharmaceuticals AB. Last updated on the eMC 22/3/2019.

SmPC from the eMC. Labetalol 100mg tablets. Generics UK T/A Mylan. Last updated on the eMC 25/5/2017.

SmPC from the eMC. Hydralazine 25mg tablets. ADVANZ Pharma. Last updated on the eMC 23/4/2014.

SmPC from the eMC. Methyldopa 250mg tablets. Intrapharm Laboratories Limited. Last updated on the eMC 31/1/2019.

SmPC from the eMC. Trandate® 100 mg film-coated tablets. RPH Pharmaceuticals AB. Last updated on the eMC 25/3/2019.

Webster, S., Dodd, C., & Waugh, J. (2013). Hypertensive Disorders. In E. Robson, & J. Waugh (Eds.), *Medical Disorders in Pregnancy: A Manual for Midwives* (2nd ed.). Chichester, WSussex: Wiley Blackwell.

Webster, S., & Waugh, J. (2017). Hypertension in pregnancy. In D. James, P. Steer, C. Weiner, B. Gonik, & S. Robson (Eds.), *High Risk Pregnancy: Management Options* (5th ed.) (pp. 847–899). Cambridge: Cambridge University Press.

Weiner, C., & Mason, C. (2017). Medication. In D. James, P. Steer, C. Weiner, B. Gonik, & S. Robson (Eds.), *High Risk Pregnancy: Management Options* (5th ed.) (pp. 808–846). Cambridge: Cambridge University Press.

12

Antiseptics

These substances are also known as disinfectants, bacteriostats, bactericides and germicides. They inhibit the growth of, or kill, microorganisms. Antiseptics are usually applied to the body or as disinfectants to equipment, etc. Skin cleansers are also included in this chapter.

The student should be aware of:

- the difference between antiseptics and antibiotics
- local Trust guidance for infection prevention and infection control including the promotion of good hygiene principles in all settings
- professional responsibility to promote strategies of antibiotic stewardship for women and families, e.g. compliance with prescribed antibiotic regimes, health lifestyles.

BP
Surgical alcohol (Isopropyl alcohol)

Proprietary

Sterets® (Mölnlycke Health Care AB)

Group
Alcohol-based cleanser

Uses/indications
Preparation of the skin prior to injection

Type of drug
GSL

Presentation
Injection swabs

Dosage
N/A

Route of admin
Topical

Contraindications
Broken skin, patients with burns, prior to using diathermy

Side effects
Flammable, skin irritation

Interactions
N/A

Pharmacodynamic properties
Seventy percent Isopropyl alcohol has disinfectant properties and, when used in combination with chlorhexidine, has antimicrobial qualities; therefore, it is used to clean the skin and reduce the bacteriological count prior to injection or surgery

Fetal risk
N/A

Breastfeeding
N/A

BP
Sodium chloride

Proprietary

Sodium chloride (Pfizer Limited)
Saline Steripods (Galen Limited)
Sodium chloride (non-proprietary, see BNF for details)

Group
Saline skin cleanser

Type of drug
POM

Uses/indications
Cleansing of skin and wounds

Presentation
Sterile solution in 18.5 mL and 50 mL vials or 2.5 mL hermetically sealed translucent plastic ampoules (steripods)

Dosage
N/A

Route of admin
Topical

Contraindications
N/A

Side effects
N/A

Interactions
N/A

Fetal risk
N/A

Breastfeeding
N/A

BP
Povidone–Iodine

Proprietary

Videne® surgical scrub (Ecolab Health Division)
Betadine® dry-powder spray (Aspire Pharma Ltd)

Group
Antiseptic – iodine compounds

Uses/indications
Skin disinfection, preoperative and postoperative, caution with diathermy

Type of drug
P – 7.5% surgical scrub, GSL – 10% surgical scrub
and dry powder

Presentation
Prepared solutions, powder

Dosage
N/A

Route of admin
Topical

Contraindications
Iodine sensitivity, renal impairment, regular use in
patients or users with thyroid disorders

Side effects
Sensitivity

Interactions
N/A

Pharmacodynamic properties
The povidone–iodine slowly liberates iodine on contact with the skin and mucous membranes, and acts
as a microbicide, effectively 'suffocating' the microbe
by displacing its oxygen supply and altering the stability of the microbial cell membrane

Fetal risk
Avoid regular use in pregnancy and lactation, as iodine compounds cross the placenta – may affect fetal
thyroid function in second and third trimesters

Breastfeeding
Iodine compounds are excreted in breast milk, and
although no adverse effects have been reported it
should be considered hazardous and the possible benefits should be weighed against the risks of thyroid
dysfunction and maldevelopment; avoid use on very
low birthweight babies

BP
Chlorhexidine gluconate

Proprietary

Hibiscrub® (Mölnlycke Health Care)
HiBiLiquid® handrub (Mölnlycke Health Care)
Hibitane® Obstetric Cream (Derma UK Ltd)
Chlorhexidine (non-proprietary, see BNF for details)

Group
Antiseptic – chlorhexidine salts, phenyl derivative

Uses/indications
Skin preparation prior to surgery, cleansing of perineum and vulva, lubrication of the midwife's hands (as Hibitane® Obstetric cream – chlorhexidine gluconate 1% solution in water as lubricant)

Type of drug
GSL

Presentation
Prepared solutions of varying concentrations

Dosage
N/A

Route of admin
Topical

Contraindications
Hypersensitivity, avoid contact with the eyes, brain meninges and middle ear; not suitable before diathermy

Side effects
Sensitivity

Interactions
N/A

Pharmacodynamic properties

Wide range of antimicrobial activities against Gram-positive and Gram-negative vegetative bacteria, dermatological fungi and lipophilic viruses. It is inactive against bacterial spores except at raised temperatures. Its cationic nature means that it binds strongly to skin, mucosa and other tissues, and is very poorly absorbed; therefore there are no detectable levels after oral or skin contact

Fetal risk
N/A

Breastfeeding
Considered safe (when used as a handwash)

BP
Chlorhexidine gluconate and Cetrimide solution

Proprietary
Chlorhexidine Acetate and Cetrimide [Savlon®] (Baxter Healthcare Ltd)

Group
Antiseptic – phenyl derivative and disinfectant

Uses/indications
General-purpose antiseptic, disinfectant and detergent

Type of drug
P

Presentation solution is a clear, yellow, sterile, aqueous solution for general topical use
Liquid – Chlorhexidine Acetate 0.015% w/v and Cetrimide 0.15% w/v, for irrigation of skin areas

Dosage
As instructed

Continued

Route of admin
Topical – diluted for external use only

Contraindications
Sensitivity

Side effects
Contamination by *Pseudomonas aeruginosa* – store as sterile solutions in pour bottles; keep out of eyes and ears

Interactions
N/A

Fetal risk
N/A

Breastfeeding
N/A

References and Recommended Reading

Dougherty, L., Lister, S., & West-Oram, A. (2015). *The Royal Marsden Manual of Clinical Nursing Procedures (Royal Marsden Manual Series) professional edition* (9th ed.). Chichester, West Sussex: Wiley Blackwell.

Furber, C., Allison, D., & Hindley, C. (2017). Antimicrobial resistance, antibiotic stewardship, and the midwife's role. *British Journal of Midwifery*, 25(11), 693–698.

Johnson, R., & Taylor, W. (2016). *Skills for midwifery practice* (4th ed.). Edinburgh: Elsevier.

Haas, D., Morgan, S., Contreras, K., & Enders, S. (2018). Vaginal preparation with antiseptic solution before cesarean section for preventing postoperative infections. *Cochrane Database of Systematic Reviews* (Issue 7). Available from: https://www.cochranelibrary.com/cdsr/doi/10.1002/14651858.CD007892.pub6/full. [Accessed 4 July 2019].

HiBiLiquid® handrub 0.5% solution. Mölnlycke Health Care. Last updated on the BNF [online] April 2019.

Hibiscrub® 4% solution. Mölnlycke Health Care. Last updated on the BNF [online] April 2019.

Hibitane® 1% Obstetric cream. Derma UK Ltd. Last updated on the BNF [online] April 2019.

National Institute of Health and Care Excellence (NICE). (2012). *CG 139 Healthcare-associated infections: prevention and control in primary and community care.* Last updated February 2017. Available from: https://www.nice.org.uk/guidance/cg139. [Accessed 4 July 2019].

National Institute of Health and Care Excellence (NICE). (2015). *NG15 Antimicrobial stewardship: systems and processes for effective antimicrobial medicine use.* Last updated January 2018. Available from: https://www.nice.org.uk/guidance/ng15. [Accessed 4 July 2019].

National Institute of Health and Care Excellence (NICE). (2016). *QS121 Antimicrobial stewardship.* Available from: https://www.nice.org.uk/guidance/qs121. [Accessed 4 July 2019].

Nursing and Midwifery Council (NMC), 2019. *Standards of proficiency for midwives* London: NMC. Available from: https://www.nmc.org.uk/globalassets/sitedocuments/standards/standards-of-proficiency-for-midwives.pdf. [Accessed 20 November 2019].

Otter, J., & Galletly, T. (2018). Environmental decontamination 1: What is it and why is it important? *Nursing Times, 114*(7), 32–34.

SmPC from the eMC. Betadine® dry powder spray. Aspire Pharma Ltd. Last updated on the eMC 26/1/2017.

SmPC from the eMC. Chlorhexidine acetate 0.015% and Cetrimide 0.15% for irrigation (Savlon®). Baxter Healthcare Ltd. Last updated on the eMC 29/9/2016.

SmPC from the eMC. Sodium chloride 0.9% for injection. Pfizer Limited Last updated on eMC 9/11/2016.

SmPC from the eMC. Saline 2.5 mL steripods. Galen Limited. Last updated on the eMC 22/11/2017.

Sterets® Pre-Injection Swabs with 70% Isopropyl Alcohol. Mölnlycke Health Care AB. Available from: https://www.algeos.com/sterets-pre-injection-swabs-with-70-isopropyl-alcohol---100-pack.html or https://www.medisave.co.uk/sterets-pre-injection-swabs-box-of-100.html [Accessed 20 May 2019].

Videne® surgical scrub (Povidine Iodine) 7.5% surgical scrub and 10% surgical scrub. Last updated on the BNF [online] April 2019.

Anxiolytics and Hypnotics

These are used to lessen tension and excitement and to induce sleep. They may be prescribed for anxious patients or those unable to sleep in the antenatal period during hospitalization.

The student should be aware of:

- the effects that tension has in exacerbating certain conditions
- the addictive qualities of such preparations.

BP
Temazepam

Proprietary
Temazepam (Accord-UK Ltd)
Temazepam (non-proprietary, see BNF for details)

Group
Hypnotic – benzodiazepine – shorter acting than diazepam

Uses/indications
Insomnia – short-term use only – see BNF [online] 2019

Type of drug
POM

Presentation
Tablets (white), oral solution

Dosage
10–20 mg nocte (BNF 2019)

Route of admin
Oral

Contraindications
Any history of drug/alcohol abuse including benzodi-azepine dependency, respiratory disease, myasthenia gravis, marked personality disorders, hypersensitivity to this or benzodiazepines, renal/hepatic disorder, sleep apnoea, muscle weakness

Side effects
Drowsiness, lightheadedness, reduced alertness, con-fusion, fatigue, muscle weakness, numbed emotion, headache, ataxia, double vision

Interactions
Alcohol, Analgesics, Anaesthetics, Antiepileptics, Antihistamines, Antihypertensives – all enhance the sedative effect
Antihistamines – concomitant administration with diphenhydramine can cause intrauterine or early neonatal death

Pharmacodynamic properties
A hypnotic/sedative/anxiolytic results in anxiolysis, muscle relaxation, CNS sedation, possibly acting on GABA receptors to potentiate GABA effects

Fetal risk
Associated with microcephaly and cleft palate if taken during first trimester. Drowsiness; with large doses hypotonia; during last phase of pregnancy or during labour – depression of neonatal respiration, hypother-mia and withdrawal symptoms

Breastfeeding
Considered moderately safe but avoid repeated doses – can lead to lethargy and weight loss in the infant

References and Recommended Reading

Berlin, C. (2013). Medications and the breastfeeding mother. In D. Mattison (Ed.), *Clinical pharmacology during pregnancy* (pp. 41–54). Edinburgh: Elsevier.

Briggs, G., Freeman, R., Towers, C., & Forinash, A. (2017). *Drugs in pregnancy and lactation: a reference guide to fetal and neonatal risk* (11th ed.). Philadelphia: Wolters Kluwer.

British National Formulary (BNF). (2019). *Temazepam [online]*. Available from: https://www.drugs.com/ppa/temazepam.html; https://bnf.nice.org.uk/drug/temazepam.html. [Accessed 5 July 2019].

Herbert, M. (2013). Impact of pregnancy on maternal pharmacokinetics of medications. In D. Mattison (Ed.), *Clinical pharmacology during pregnancy* (pp. 17–40). Edinburgh: Elsevier.

Jordan, S. (2010). *Pharmacology for midwives: The evidence base for safe practice* (2nd ed.). Basingstoke: Palgrave Macmillan.

Jordan, S., & MacDonald, S. (2017). Pharmacology and the midwife. In S. MacDonald, & G. Johnson (Eds.), *Mayes' midwifery: A text book for midwives* (15th ed.) (pp. 158–174). Edinburgh: Elsevier.

National Institute of Health and Care Excellence (NICE). (2008). *CG62. Antenatal care for uncomplicated pregnancies [online]*. Last updated: February 2019. London: NICE. Available from: https://www.nice.org.uk/guidance/cg62. [Accessed 4 April 2019].

Nursing and Midwifery Council (NMC). (2015). update 2018. *The code - professional standards of practice and behaviour for nurses, midwives and nursing associates*. London: NMC.

Nursing and Midwifery Council (NMC). (2017). *updated 2019. Practicing as a midwife in the UK*. London: NMC.

Nursing and Midwifery Council (NMC). (2019). *Standards of proficiency for midwives*. London: NMC. Available from: https://www.nmc.org.uk/globalassets/sitedocuments/standards/standards-of-proficiency-for-midwives.pdf . [Accessed 20 April 2019].

SmPC from the eMC. Temazepam 10mg and 20mg tablets. Accord-UK Ltd. Last updated on the eMC 23/11/2018.

SmPC from the eMC. Temazepam 10mg/5ml oral solution. Rosemont Pharmaceuticals Limited. Last updated on the eMC 21/9/2016.

Weiner, C., & Mason, C. (2017). Medication. In D. James, P. Steer, C. Weiner, B. Gonik, & S. Robson (Eds.), *High risk pregnancy: Management options* (5th ed.) (pp. 808–846). Cambridge: Cambridge University Press.

14

Contraceptives

This is a general term to describe an agent used to prevent conception.

As part of their sphere of practice, midwives have a duty to offer family planning advice (Nursing and Midwifery Council [NMC] 2012; NICE 2006; Article 42 of the European Union Standards for Nursing and Midwifery [WHO 2009]).

The student should be aware of:

- the availability of contraception (hormonal, intrauterine devices, barrier methods, spermicidal and emergency contraception)
- the importance of family planning
- the process of contraception with a view to usage of emergency contraception
- the appropriateness of the contraceptive prescribed
- the importance of counselling – advice on bleeding, missed pills, diarrhoea and vomiting, antibiotic administration, and cessation of oral contraception prior to surgery.

BP

Combined oestrogen–progestogen oral contraceptive (COC)

Proprietary

Femodene® (Bayer PLC)
Loestrin 20® and Loestrin 30® (Galen Ltd)
Marvelon® (Merck Sharp & Dohme Ltd)
Microgynon 30® ED (Bayer PLC)
Millinette® 20/75 mcg (Consilient Health Ltd)
Ovranette® 150/30 mcg (Pfizer Ltd)
Yasmin® 0.03 mg/3 mg (Bayer PLC)

Continued

Group

Contraceptive – hormonal; combinations of two of the following: ethinylestradiol, desogestrel, levonorgestrel, drospirenone, norgestimate

Uses/indications

Contraception, menstrual symptoms

Type of drug

POM

Presentation

Tablets in packs for 1 month, with days numbered

Dosage

Usually 1 tablet/day, but refer to pack for instructions

Postpartum (not breastfeeding) – commence at 3 weeks' postpartum – there is an increased risk of DVT if commenced earlier – patient must be fully ambulant, with no puerperal complications, and be counselled for the risk of DVT

Breastfeeding – not recommended until weaning or at least 6 months if unable to obtain other contraception

Miscarriage or abortion – commence on same day if possible

Route of admin

Oral

Contraindications

Pregnancy, migraine, liver disease including cholestatic jaundice, history of pruritus in pregnancy, breastfeeding, prothrombotic coagulation disorders, previous history or strong familial history of DVT, undiagnosed vaginal bleeding, breast or genital tract carcinoma

CAUTION: arterial disease, smoking, hypertension, obesity, diabetes mellitus with retinopathy and nephropathy, ischaemic heart disease, varicosities, depression, inflammatory bowel disease, Rotor syndrome, Dubin–Johnson syndrome, sickle cell anaemia, history of herpes gestationis, disorders of lipid metabolism

Stop prior to major surgery or surgery to the legs, or with long-term immobilization – do not stop for minor surgery with short anaesthetic duration, e.g. laparoscopy or tooth extraction

Side effects

Nausea, vomiting, headache, breast tenderness, changes in body weight, libido changes, DVT, intracycle bleeding, amenorrhoea, decreased menstrual bleeding, depression, impaired liver function

Interactions

Antibiotics – broad spectrum – reduce effect

Anticoagulants – antagonizes the effect of warfarin

Antidepressants – tricyclics – antagonizes the antidepressant effects but increases the side effects because of the increased plasma concentration of tricyclics

Antidiabetics – antagonism of the hypoglycaemic effect

Antiepileptics – carbamazepine, phenobarbital and phenytoin accelerate metabolism and reduce contraceptive effect

Antihypertensives – antagonize hypotensive effect

Pharmacodynamic properties

The combination of these preparations acts to inhibit ovulation by suppressing the mid-cycle surge of luteinizing hormone, thickening the cervical mucus as a barrier to sperm, and rendering the endometrium unresponsive to implantation

Fetal risk

Evidence suggests no harmful effects to fetus, although there is teratogenicity in animals (US studies have found a small risk of 0.07% of all pregnancies exposed to the oral contraceptive pill)

Breastfeeding

Suppresses lactation; contraindicated until at least 6 months after birth (weaning)

Continued

BP
Progestogen-only pill (POP)

Proprietary
Cerazette® 75 mcg (Merck Sharp & Dohme Ltd)
Cerelle 75 mcg (Consilient Health Ltd)
Desogestrel 75 mcg (Accord-UK Ltd)
Feanolla 75 mcg (Lupin Healthcare (UK))
Norgeston® (Bayer PLC)
Noriday® (Pfizer Ltd)

Group
Contraceptive – hormonal; levonorgestrel, desogestrel

Uses/indications
Contraception, alternative to oestrogens – higher failure rate, suitable in smokers, hypertension, valvular heart disease, diabetes mellitus, migraine, predisposition to or history of thrombosis or venous thrombosis

Type of drug
POM

Presentation
Tablets in cyclical packs

Dosage
Usually 1 tablet/day, but refer to pack instructions – must be taken at the same time each day postpartum – commence after 3 weeks – breakthrough bleeding if earlier – women should also be aware of the increased risk of thromboembolic disorders

Route of admin
Oral

Contraindications
Pregnancy, undiagnosed vaginal bleeding, severe arterial disease, existing thrombophlebitis or thromboembolic disorders, cerebrovascular disease, porphyria,

heart disease including myocardial infarction, malabsorption syndromes, liver disease, sex steroid-dependent cancers, past ectopic pregnancy, functional ovarian cysts, cholestatic jaundice, pruritus of pregnancy, Dubin–Johnson syndrome, Rotor syndrome, history of herpes gestationis, disorders of lipid metabolism

Side effects
Menstrual irregularities, nausea, vomiting, menstrual symptoms, weight change, depression, dizziness, loss of libido, headaches, chloasma

Interactions
Antibiotics – rifamycins – increase metabolism and therefore reduce effect
Anticoagulants – antagonize effect of warfarin
Antidiabetics – antagonize the hypoglycaemic effects
Antiepileptics – reduce contraceptive effect
St John's wort – can lead to potential loss of contraceptive effect

Pharmacodynamic properties
POPs have a progestational effect on the endometrium and cervical mucus that discourages implantation and decreases corpus luteum function

Fetal risk
High doses may be teratogenic in the first trimester (US studies have found a 0.07 % risk) and cause masculinization of the fetus, although only with very high progestogen doses

Breastfeeding
Not contraindicated, but not before 3 weeks' postpartum
Manufacturer advises avoidance, as small amounts of active ingredients are excreted in breast milk and the effects on the infant are unknown

Continued

BP
Etonogestrel

Proprietary
Nexplanon® (Merck Sharp & Dohme Ltd)

Group
Parenteral progestogen-only contraceptive;
etonogestrel

Uses/indications
Contraception effective for up to 3 years – rapidly
reversible on removal

Type of drug
POM

Presentation
Non-biodegradable white to off-white flexible rod –
for subdermal use

Dosage
68 mg etonogestrel in each rod with no previous hormonal contraception: one implant in the first 5 days of
the cycle (eMC 7/3/2019)
Parturition/abortion in second trimester: 1 implant
21–28 days after delivery or abortion

Route of admin
Subdermal

Contraindications
As for progestogen-only pill

Side effects
Aching, pain at site, tiredness, acne, alopecia,
headache, dizziness, depression, mood swings,
libido changes, gastrointestinal disturbances, weight
changes, menstrual symptoms, occasional hypertension, vaginal infection, acne, increased risk of DVT

Interactions
As for progestogen-only pill

Pharmacodynamic properties

A progestogen that inhibits progesterone receptors in target organs

Primarily it works to inhibit ovulation, and also to thicken the cervical mucus, making it hostile to spermatozoa

Fetal risk

As for progestogen-only pill

Breastfeeding

As for progestogen-only pill

BP

Medroxyprogesterone acetate

Proprietary

Depo-Provera® injection (Pfizer Ltd)

Group

Parenteral progesterone-only contraceptive; medroxyprogesterone acetate

Uses/indications

Depo-Provera is a long-term contraceptive agent suitable for use in women who have been appropriately counselled concerning the likelihood of menstrual disturbance and the potential for a delay in return to full fertility. Depo-Provera may also be used for short-term contraception in the following circumstances:

- for partners of men undergoing vasectomy, for protection until the vasectomy becomes effective
- in women who are being immunized against rubella, to prevent pregnancy during the period of activity of the virus
- in women awaiting sterilization

Type of drug

POM

Continued

Presentation
Aqueous suspension in vials

Dosage
150 mg in first 5 days of menstrual cycle or within 5 days of parturition; repeat in 12 weeks (eMC 12/2/2019)

Route of admin
IM

Contraindications
As for progestogen-only preparations; use reduces serum oestrogen levels and is associated with significant loss of bone mass density due to the effect of oestrogen deficiency on the bone remodelling; bone loss is greater with increasing duration of use but reduces when discontinued

Side effects
Common side effects: menstrual irregularities (bleeding and/or amenorrhoea), weight changes, headache, nervousness, abdominal pain or discomfort, dizziness, asthenia (weakness or fatigue); adverse events reported by 1–5%: decreased libido or anorgasmia, backache, leg cramps, depression, nausea, insomnia, leucorrhoea, acne, vaginitis, pelvic pain, breast pain, no hair growth or alopecia, bloating, rash, oedema, hot flushes

Interactions
As for progestogen-only preparations

Pharmacodynamic properties
Exerts an antiandrogenic and antigonadotrophic effect that inhibits ovulation and endometrial preparation for pregnancy

Fetal risk
Possible increase in low birthweight that is associated with increased risk of neonatal death – although the attributable risk is low as pregnancies are uncommon; those exposed show no adverse effects

Breastfeeding
Secreted into breast milk but no evidence of harmful effects; may be advised to withhold for the first 6 weeks postnatally if breastfeeding

BP
Norethisterone enanthate

Proprietary
Noristerat® injection (Bayer PLC)

Group
Parenteral progestogen-only contraceptive

Uses/indications
Short-term or interim contraception, 8 weeks' duration

Type of drug
POM

Presentation
Oily preparation in ampoules

Dosage
Deep IM: 200 mg in first 5 days of cycle or immediately after parturition; repeat in 8 weeks (eMC 15/2/2018)

Route of admin
Deep IM

Contraindications
As for progestogen-only preparations

Side effects
As for progestogen-only preparations

Interactions
As for progestogen-only preparations

Fetal risk
As for progestogen-only preparations

Continued

Breastfeeding
Withhold when neonate has severe jaundice requiring medical treatment; may also suppress lactation in high doses and alter composition of breast milk, therefore use the lowest effective dose

BP
Levonorgestrel

Proprietary
Levonelle® One Step (Bayer PLC)

Group
Emergency contraception

Uses/indications
Emergency contraception within 72 hours (3 days) of unprotected sexual intercourse or failure of a contraceptive method

Type of drug
P (over 16 years of age by pharmacists only)

Presentation
Tablets

Dosage
1 tablet (1500 mcg levonorgestrel) should be taken as soon as possible, preferably within 12 hours and no later than 72 hours after unprotected intercourse (eMC 21/6/2018)

Route of admin
Oral

Contraindications
Pregnancy, porphyria, overdue menstrual bleeding or unprotected intercourse more than 72 hours previously, bowel disease, liver disease, history of ectopic pregnancy, salpingitis, and the use of some other medications

Side effects
Nausea, abdominal pain, vomiting, headache, fatigue, breast discomfort

Interactions
The metabolism of levonorgestrel is enhanced by concomitant use of liver enzyme inducers Possible drugs suspected of reducing the efficacy of levonorgestrel-containing medication include barbiturates (including primidone), phenytoin, carbamazepine, herbal medicines containing *Hypericum perforatum* (St John's wort), rifampicin, ritonavir, rifabutin, griseofulvin
Women taking such drugs should be referred to their doctor for advice

Pharmacodynamic properties
Inhibits ovulation if taken in the pre-ovulatory stage, and also causes endometrial changes that discourage implantation; however, once implantation has occurred it is no longer an effective contraceptive
It is effective in up to 84% when given within 72 hours of intercourse (3 days)

Fetal risk
Abortifacient, but pregnancy may continue; monitor for signs of ectopic pregnancy
In theory, because there is no organogenesis at 72 hours there should be no teratogenicity

Breastfeeding
Exposure of the infant is reduced if the mother avoids nursing post medication

References and Recommended Reading

Berlin, C. (2013). Medications and the breastfeeding mother. In D. Mattison (Ed.), *Clinical pharmacology during pregnancy* (pp. 41–54). Edinburgh: Elsevier.

Briggs, G., Freeman, R., Towers, C., & Forinash, A. (2017). *Drugs in Pregnancy and Lactation: A reference guide to fetal and neonatal risk* (11th ed.). Philadelphia: Wolters Kluwer.

Hall, J. (2017). Fertility and its control. In S. Macdonald, & G. Johnson (Eds.), *Mayes' Midwifery* (15th ed.) (pp. 413–425). Edinburgh: Elsevier.

Jackson, K. (2017). Contraception and sexual health in a global society. In J. Marshall, & M. Raynor (Eds.), *Myles textbook for midwives* (16th ed.) (pp. 569–589). Edinburgh: Churchill Livingstone.

Jordan, S. (Ed.). (2010). *Pharmacology for Midwives: The Evidence Base for Safe Practice* (2nd ed.) Basingstoke: Palgrave Macmillan.

National Institute of Health and Care Excellence (NICE). (2006). *CG37. Postnatal care up to 8 weeks after birth [online]*. Last updated February 2015. London: NICE. Available from: https://www.nice.org.uk/guidanc e/cg37. [Accessed 14 April 2019].

Nursing and Midwifery Council (NMC). (2012). *Midwives Rules and Standards*. London: NMC.

Nursing and Midwifery Council (NMC). (2015). *The Code for Nurses and Midwives [online]*. London: NMC. Available from: https://www.nm c.org.uk/standards/code/. [Accessed 17 May 2017].

Nursing and Midwifery Council (NMC). (2019). *Standards of proficiency for midwives*. London: NMC. Available from: https://www.nmc.org. uk/globalassets/sitedocuments/standards/standards-of-proficiency-for-midwives.pdf [Accessed 20 November 2019].

SmPC from the eMC. Brevinor® tablets. Pfizer Ltd. Last updated on the eMC 4/4/2019.

SmPC from the eMC. Cerazette® 75 mcg tablets. Merck Sharp & Dohme Ltd. Last updated on the eMC 25/2/2019.

SmPC from the eMC. Cerrelle® 75 mcg tablets. Consilient Health Ltd. Last updated on the eMC 25/3/2019.

SmPC from the eMC. Cilest® 35/250 mcg tablets. Janssen-Cilag Ltd. Last updated on the eMC 7/2/2019.

SmPC from the eMC. Depo-Provera® 150mg/mL injection. Pfizer Ltd. Last updated on the eMC 20/2/2019.

SmPC from the eMC. Desogestrel® 75 microgram tablets. Accord-UK Ltd. Last updated on the eMC 24/9/2015.

SmPC from the eMC. Feanolla® 75 microgram tablets. Lupin Health-care (UK). Last updated on the eMC 7/10/2015.

SmPC from the eMC. Femedene® tablets. Bayer PLC. Last updated on the eMC 1/1/2019.

SmPC from the eMC. Levonell® one step. Bayer PLC. Last updated on the eMC 21/6/2018.

SmPC from the eMC. Loestrin® 20 and 30 tablets. Galen Ltd. Last updated on the eMC12/2/2019.

SmPC from the eMC. Marvelon® tablets. Merck Sharp & Dohme Ltd. Last updated on the eMC 25/1/2019.

SmPC from the eMC. Microgynon® 30 and 30ED tablets. Bayer PLC. Last updated on the eMC 4/2/2019.

SmPC from the eMC. Millinette® 20/75 mcg tablets. Consilient Health Ltd. Last updated on the eMC 2/10/2017.

SmPC from the eMC. Nexplanon® 68mg implant. Merck Sharp & Dohme Ltd. Last updated on the eMC 7/3/2019.

SmPC from the eMC. Noristerat® 200mg injection. Bayer PLC. Last updated on the eMC 15/2/2018.

SmPC from the eMC. Norgeston® tablets. Bayer PLC. Last updated on the eMC 4/2/2019.

SmPC from the eMC. Noriday® tablets. Pfizer. Last updated on the eMC 28/1/2019.

SmPC from the eMC. Ovrentette® 150/30 mcg tablets. Pfizer Ltd. Last updated on the eMC 11/4/2019.

SmPC from the eMC. Yasmin® 0.03mg/3mg tablets. Bayer PLC. Last updated on the eMC 6/3/2019.

Weiner, C., & Mason, C. (2017). Medication. In D. James, P. Steer, C. Weiner, B. Gonik, & S. Robson (Eds.), *High Risk Pregnancy: Management Options* (5th ed.) (pp. 808–846). Cambridge: Cambridge University Press.

World Health Organization. (2009). *European Union Standard for Nursing and Midwifery: Information for Accession Countries*. Available http://www.euro.who.int/__data/assets/pdf_file/0005/102200/E92852.pdf. [Accessed 14 April 2019].

15

Emergency Drugs

This chapter includes some of the drugs used in emergencies such as cardiac arrest, anaphylaxis and eclampsia. See also Chapters 18 and 21 for medications used for haemorrhage.

The new standards for proficiency for midwives have been published (NMC 2019). In the event of emergency situations or clinical complications, student midwives will need to demonstrate specific proficiencies for safe medicines administration and optimisation when working collaboratively with a range of professionals (NMC 2019 p48). Each student should quickly become familiar with the local protocols and policies that cover such emergencies and seek adequate training in resuscitation techniques.

Drugs Used in the Treatment of Cardiac Arrest

Cardiac arrest may be associated with ventricular fibrillation, pulseless ventricular tachycardia, asystole and pulseless electrical activity (electromechanical dissociation).

BP
Adrenaline (epinephrine)

Proprietary

Cardiac arrest
Adrenaline (Epinephrine) 1 : 10 000 Sterile Solution (Martindale Pharma)
Anaphylaxis
Adrenaline (Epinephrine) Injection BP 1 : 1000 (Martindale Pharma)

Group

Cardiopulmonary resuscitation, allergic emergencies

Uses/indications

Asystolic cardiac arrest in conjunction with calcium chloride and defibrillation. Increases cardiac output and force of contractility by producing generalized vasoconstriction by acting on vascular smooth muscle **anaphylactic shock** or severe allergic reactions

Type of drug

POM, Midwives' Exemptions

Presentation

Ampoules, auto-injector, pre-filled pen, pre-filled syringe

Dosage

Cardiac arrest:

Adrenaline (Epinephrine) 1 : 10 000:

- 10 mL (1 mg) by IV injection repeated every 3–5 minutes as necessary (eMC 20/4/2018)
- or if venous access if difficult or impossible, the intraosseous (IO) route may be used

Sodium Chloride 0.9% injection: 20 mL peripherally must be administered following adrenaline to aid entry into the central circulation (BNF [online] June 2019)

Anaphylactic shock:

Adrenaline Injection BP 1/1000: 500 mcg (0.5 mL adrenaline 1/1000). May be repeated several times at 5-min intervals according to blood pressure, pulse and respiratory function (eMC 20/12/2017)

Route of admin

Cardiac arrest:

Adrenaline (Ephedrine) 1 : 10 000 – IV (if administered via a central line must not interrupt CPR), intracardiac injection or intraosseous route

Anaphylaxis:

Adrenaline Injection BP 1/1000 – S.C./IM/IV (UK Resuscitation Council (2015) recommends IM)

NB: the needle used needs to be long enough to ensure that adrenaline is injected into the muscle; IV use restricted to specialists

Contraindications

Cardiac arrest: Adrenaline (Epinephrine) 1 : 10 000

Contraindications are relative as this product is intended for use in life-threatening emergencies

Other than in the emergency situation, the following contraindications should be considered: hyperthyroidism, hypertension, ischaemic heart disease, diabetes mellitus and closed-angle glaucoma

Anaphylaxis: Adrenaline Injection BP 1/1000

Use during labour

With local anaesthesia of peripheral structures including digits, ear lobe

In the presence of ventricular fibrillation, cardiac dilatation, coronary insufficiency, organic brain disease or atherosclerosis, except in emergencies where the potential benefit clearly outweighs the risk

If the solution is discoloured

Side effects

Ventricular fibrillation may occur and severe hypertension may lead to cerebral haemorrhage and pulmonary oedema

Symptomatic adverse effects are anxiety, dyspnoea, restlessness, palpitations, tachycardia, anginal pain, tremor, weakness, dizziness, headache and cold extremities

Biochemical effects include inhibition of insulin secretion, stimulation of growth hormone secretion, hyperglycaemia (even with low doses), gluconeogenesis, glycolysis, lipolysis and ketogenesis

Interactions

The effects of adrenaline may be potentiated by **tricyclic antidepressants**

Volatile **liquid anaesthetics** such as halothane increase the risk of adrenaline-induced ventricular arrhythmias and acute pulmonary oedema if hypoxia is present

Severe hypertension and bradycardia may occur with non-selective β-blocking drugs such as propranolol Propranolol also inhibits the bronchodilator effect of adrenaline

Risk of cardiac arrhythmias is higher when adrenaline is given to patients receiving **digoxin** or **quinidine**

Risk of hypertensive crisis with **MAOIs**

Adrenaline-induced hyperglycaemia may lead to loss of blood-sugar control in diabetic patients treated with **hypoglycaemic agents**

The vasoconstrictor and pressor effects of adrenaline, mediated by its α-adrenergic action, may be enhanced by concomitant administration of drugs with similar effects, such as **ergot alkaloids** or **oxytocin**

Adrenaline specifically reverses the antihypertensive effects of **adrenergic neurone blockers** with the risk of severe hypertension

Pharmacodynamic properties

Adrenaline is a naturally occurring catecholamine secreted by the adrenal medulla in response to exertion or stress. It is a sympathomimetic amine and a potent stimulant of both α- and β-adrenergic receptors

Rapid relief of hypersensitivity reactions to allergies or to idiopathic or exercise-induced anaphylaxis

Has a strong vasoconstrictor action through α-adrenergic stimulation, which counteracts the vasodilatation and increased vascular permeability leading to loss of intravascular fluid and subsequent hypotension, the major features in anaphylactic shock

Continued

Stimulates bronchial β-adrenergic receptors and has a powerful bronchodilator action

Alleviates pruritus, urticaria and angio-oedema associated with anaphylaxis

In resuscitation procedures it is used to increase the efficacy of basic life support

Increased systolic blood pressure, reduced diastolic pressure (increased at higher doses), tachycardia, hyperglycaemia and hypokalaemia

Fetal risk

Crosses the placenta. There is some evidence of a slightly increased incidence of congenital abnormalities

Injection of adrenaline may cause anoxia, fetal tachycardia, cardiac irregularities, extrasystoles and louder heart sounds

Usually inhibits spontaneous or oxytocin-induced contractions of the uterus and may delay the second stage of labour; if uterine contractions are reduced there may be uterine atony with haemorrhage

Parenteral adrenaline should not be used during the second stage of labour

Breastfeeding

Secreted in breast milk and should be avoided

BP

Amiodarone hydrochloride

Proprietary

Amiodarone Hydrochloride (hameln pharmaceuticals Ltd)
Amiodarone Injection (Martindale Pharma), amiodarone (non-proprietary, see BNF for details)

Group

Cardiac arrhythmias

Uses/indications
Severe rhythm disorders not responding to
other therapies or when other treatments cannot
be used

Type of drug
POM

Presentation
Solution for injection

Dosage
IV amiodarone 300 mg (from a pre-filled syringe or
diluted in 20 mL glucose 5%) should be considered
after adrenaline to treat ventricular fibrillation or
pulseless ventricular tachycardia in cardiac arrest
refractory to defibrillation (eMC 10/1/2019)
An additional dose of amiodarone 150 mg can be
given by IV injection if necessary, followed by an IV
infusion of amiodarone 900 mg over 24 hours (BNF
[online] June 2019)

Route of admin
IV

Contraindications
Hypersensitivity to any of the excipients, e.g.
iodine
Infants and children up to 3 years old
Severe respiratory failure, circulatory collapse, or
severe arterial hypotension; hypotension, heart failure
and cardiomyopathy are also contraindications if 50
mg/mL is given as a bolus injection
Evidence or history of thyroid dysfunction or cardiac
conditions
**NB: the above contraindications do not apply if
cardiac arrest**

Side effects
Infusion phlebitis, bradycardia, hypotension

Continued

Interactions

Due to the long and variable half-life of amiodarone (approximately 50 days), potential for drug interactions exists not only with concomitant medication but also with drugs administered after discontinuation of amiodarone

Warfarin, phenytoin, digoxin and any drug that prolongs the QT interval

Pharmacodynamic properties

A membrane-stabilizing antiarrhythmic drug that increases the duration of the action potential and refractory period in atrial and ventricular myocardium

Fetal risk

Crosses placental barrier

Most frequent complications include impaired growth, preterm birth and impaired function of the thyroid gland

Some evidence of hypothyroidism, bradycardia and prolonged QT intervals, increased thyroid gland or cardiac murmurs

Malformation does not appear to be increased, although cardiac defects need to be considered

Given the long half-life of amiodarone, women of childbearing age would need to plan for a pregnancy starting at least half a year after finishing therapy, in order to avoid exposure of the embryo/fetus during early pregnancy

Breastfeeding

If therapy is required during the lactation period or if taken during pregnancy, breastfeeding should be stopped

BP
Lidocaine

Proprietary

Lidocaine Hydrochloride Injection 1% (hameln pharmaceuticals Ltd)
Lidocaine (non-proprietary, see BNF for details)

Group
Cardiac arrhythmias

Uses/indications
An alternative but only if amiodarone unavailable
After acute myocardial infarction it suppresses ventricular arrhythmias and reduces the potential for fibrillation and its recurrence
It decreases myocardial contractility and arterial blood pressure, and can be used where there is persistent ventricular fibrillation or ventricular tachycardia

Presentation
Pre-filled syringe (Lidocaine Hydrochloride BP 10 mg/mL)

Dosage
100 mg as a bolus over a few minutes (reduced to 50 mg in lighter patients), followed by an infusion of 4 mg/min for 30 min, 2 mg/min for 2 hours, then 1 mg/min; reduce concentration further if infusion continued beyond 24 hours (ECG monitoring and specialist advice for infusion) (see BNF [online] June 2019 for guidance)

Route of admin
IV

Contraindications

Hypersensitivity to local anaesthetics of the amide type and in patients with porphyria
NB: continuous ECG monitoring is necessary during IV administration

Continued

Resuscitative equipment and drugs should be available immediately for the management of severe adverse cardiovascular, respiratory or central nervous system effects
CAUTION: epilepsy, liver disease, congestive heart failure, severe renal disease, marked hypoxia, severe respiratory depression, hypovolaemia or shock, and in patients with any form of heart block or sinus bradycardia; hypokalaemia, hypoxia and disorders of acid–base balance should be corrected before treatment with lidocaine begins

Side effects
Allergic reactions (including anaphylaxis)
Light-headedness, drowsiness, dizziness, apprehension, nervousness, euphoria, tinnitus, blurred or double vision, nystagmus, vomiting, sensations of heat, cold or numbness, twitching, tremors, paraesthesia, convulsions, unconsciousness, respiratory depression and arrest, hypotension, cardiovascular collapse and bradycardia which may lead to cardiac arrest

Interactions
Propranolol and cimetidine may reduce the renal and hepatic clearance of lidocaine resulting in increased toxicity. The cardiac depressant effects of lidocaine are additive to those of other antiarrhythmic agents. Lidocaine prolongs the action of suxamethonium

Pharmacodynamic properties
Reduces automaticity by decreasing the rate of diastolic (phase 4) depolarization. Lidocaine is considered as a class 1b (membrane stabilizing) antiarrhythmic agent. The duration of the action potential is reduced due to the blockade of the sodium channel and the refractory period is shortened

Fetal risk
Safety has not been established, use if benefit outweighs risk

Breastfeeding
Caution as excreted in breast milk

BP
Midazolam hydrochloride

Proprietary

Midazolam (hameln pharmaceuticals Ltd)
Midazolam hydrochloride (non-proprietary, see BNF
for details)

Group
POM

Uses/indications
Short-acting, sleep-inducing drug that is indicated
for: conscious sedation before and during diagnos-
tic or therapeutic procedures with or without local
anaesthesia, anaesthesia, pre-medication for induction
of anaesthesia, induction of anaesthesia and sedation
in intensive care. Cardiac arrest and peri-arrest (UK
Resuscitation Council 2015)

Type of drug
Hypnotic/potent sedative

Presentation
Clear, colourless solution in 1-mg, 2-mg and 5-mg
ampoules

Dosage
Must be titrated and administered very slowly.
Conscious Sedation: slow IV injection to max dose of
2–2.5 mg over 5–10 mins at a rate of 1 mg over 30
seconds. Usual total dose of 5 mg (eMC 21/1/2019)
Sedation for intensive care: 30–300 mcg/kg, dose
to be given in steps of 1–2.5 mg every 2 min, then
(by slow IV injection or by continuous IV infusion)
30–200 mcg/kg/hour (see BNF 2019 for guidance)

Continued

Route of admin
IM injection or infusion

Contraindications
Hypersensitivity to benzodiazepines or to any of the excipients. Conscious sedation in patients with severe respiratory failure or acute respiratory depression

Side effects
Anaphylactic shock, angioedema, angioedema, confusional state, involuntary movements (including tonic/clonic movements and muscle tremor), hyperactivity, dependence, withdrawal, prolonged sedation, somnolence, headache, dizziness, ataxia, anterograde amnesia, cardiac arrest, respiratory depression, apnoea, respiratory arrest, dyspnoea, laryngospasm, nausea, vomiting, constipation, dry mouth, fatigue, erythema and pain on injection site, thrombophlebitis, thrombosis, risk of falls and fractures is increased in those taking concomitant sedatives

Interactions
Fluconazole, Erythromycin and *HIV protease inhibitors* may cause an increase in plasma concentration; *rifampicin, carbamazepine or phenytoin* may decrease the plasma concentrations; *St John's wort* will decrease plasma concentrations by 20–40%; co-administration with *other sedative/hypnotic agents and CNS depressants* including alcohol, is likely to result in enhanced sedation and respiratory depression, e.g. *benzodiazepines* or *opioids* increase the risk of sedation, respiratory depression, coma and death

Pharmacodynamic properties
Sedative and sleep-inducing effect of pronounced intensity. Anxiolytic, anticonvulsant and muscle-relaxant effect. Half-life is prolonged ×6 in the critically ill

Fetal risk

Insufficient data are available but reported to produce maternal or fetal adverse effects (inhalation risk in mother, irregularities in the fetal heart rate) if administered in the last trimester of pregnancy, during labour or when used as an induction agent of anaesthesia for caesarean section

Manufacturers recommend it should not be used during pregnancy or for caesarean unless clearly necessary

Breastfeeding

Low quantities found in breast milk. Reported to be associated with hypotonia, poor sucking, hypothermia and respiratory depression in the neonate. Manufacturers advise to discontinue breastfeeding for 24 hours following administration of midazolam

Patients requiring IV sodium bicarbonate are unlikely to be fit enough to breastfeed, but recovery may alter outcome and breastfeeding could be initiated later

---

BP

Adenosine

Proprietary

Adenosine (Wockhardt UK Ltd)
Adenosine (non-proprietary, see BNF for details)

Group

Anti-arrhythmic

Uses/indications

Coronary vasodilator – rapid conversion of paroxysmal supraventricular tachycardias (SVT) to normal sinus rhythm. Indicated IV use in cardiac arrest and peri-arrest scenarios (eMC 15/6/2015)

Continued

Type of drug
POM

Presentation
Clear, colourless solution

Dosage
IV bolus injection or into IV line. Resuscitation equipment must be available for immediate use including ECG recording during administration (eMC 15/6/2015)
Cardiac arrest: 3-mg bolus over 2 seconds. If SVT not resolved in 1–2 mins, 6-mg rapid bolus. Third dose of 12 mg if SVT unresolved at further 1- to 2-min intervals. Additional doses are not recommended (see BNF 2019)

Route of admin
IV

Contraindications
Asthma; chronic obstructive lung disease, decompensated heart failure, long QT syndrome, second/third-degree AV block and sick sinus syndrome (unless pacemaker fitted) and severe hypotension

Side effects
Common: Bradycardia, sinus pause, skipped beats, atrial extrasystoles, atrio-ventricular block, ventricular excitability disorders such as ventricular extrasystoles, non-sustained ventricular tachycardia, headache, dizziness, light-headedness, dyspnea (or the urge to take a deep breath), flushing chest pressure/pain, feeling of thoracic constriction/oppression and apprehension
Rare: Atrial fibrillation, severe bradycardia not corrected by atropine and possibly requiring temporary pacing, ventricular excitability disorders including ventricular fibrillation and torsade de pointes. Transient and spontaneously rapidly reversible worsening of intracranial hypertension, bronchospasm and injection site reactions

Interactions

Dipyridamole (antiplatelet medication) inhibits adenosine cellular uptake and metabolism and potentiates the action of adenosine. *Aminophylline, theophylline* and other *xanthines* are competitive adenosine antagonists and should be avoided for 24 hours prior to use of adenosine.

Food and drinks containing *xanthines* (tea, coffee, chocolate and cola) should be avoided for at least 12 hours prior to use of adenosine injection.

Pharmacodynamic properties

Adenosine is a purine nucleoside which slows conduction through the AV node (negative dromotrophic effect). This interrupts re-entry circuits involving the AV node and restores normal sinus rhythm in patients with paroxysmal SVT. The interruption stops the tachycardia and normal sinus rhythm is re-established.

Fetal risk

There is limited research data from the use of adenosine in pregnant women. Animal studies are insufficient with respect to reproductive toxicity. Adenosine is not recommended during pregnancy unless the benefits outweigh the potential risks

Breastfeeding

It is unknown whether adenosine metabolites are excreted in human milk. Manufacturers recommend it should not be used

---

BP

Intravenous lipid emulsion (ILE)

Proprietary

Intralipid® 20% (Baxter Healthcare Ltd)

Group

Fat emulsion

Uses/indications

Antidote for severe local anesthetic systemic toxicity (LAST) or poisoning (Source http://www.lipidrescue.org/; also https://www.aagbi.org/sites/default/files/la_toxicity_notes_2010_0.pdf)

Type of drug

POM

Presentation

Emulsion (20% soybean oil, 1.2% egg yolk, phospholipids 2.25%, glycerin and water for injection) in 250 mL, and 500 mL Biofine® containers

Do not store above 25°C (77°F) or freeze; if accidentally frozen, discard the bag

Dosage

Cardiopulmonary resuscitation: if no response to standard procedures IV initial bolus 1.5 mL/kg over 1 min, then infusion of 15 mL/kg/hour (see BNF 2019 for guidance). If cardiovascular stability has not been restored or circulation deteriorates at 5 mins, give a maximum of two further bolus doses of 1.5 mL/kg over 1 min, 5 min apart, and increase the infusion rate to 30 mL/kg/h. Continue until stable and adequate circulation restored or maximum cumulative dose of 12 mL/kg is given. See Management of Severe Local Anesthetic Toxicity https://www.aagbi.org/sites/default/files/la_toxicity_2010_0.pdf and see BNF (2019)

Route of admin

IV – bolus or infusion

Contraindications

Disturbances of normal fat metabolism, e.g. pathological hyperlipemia, lipoid nephrosis or acute pancreatitis; renal disease, liver disease, pulmonary disease, anaemia and blood coagulation disorders

Side effects

Thrombophlebitis, contamination of cannula which may lead to sepsis, dyspnea, cyanosis, allergic reactions, hyperlipemia, hypercoagulability, nausea, vomiting, headache, flushing, increase in temperature, sweating, sleepiness, pain in the chest and back, slight pressure over the eyes, and dizziness

Reduced ability to eliminate transfused fats, so monitor serum triglycerides; beware of *overdose, potential of fat embolism and aluminum toxicity*

Interactions

Product contains aluminum

Pharmacodynamic properties

Local anaesthetics inhibit voltage at the cell membrane sodium channels, limiting action potential and the conduction of nerve signals. LAST can present with cardiovascular collapse that is refractory to standard resuscitative measures (Lavonas et al. 2015)

The ILE's efficacy in treating cardiotoxicity, is the "lipid sink" theory – an expanded intravascular lipid phase that acts to absorb the offending circulating lipophilic toxin, hence reducing the unbound free toxin available to bind to the myocardium (Ciechanowicz and Patil 2012)

Fetal risk

No studies available; manufacturers recommend avoidance

Breastfeeding

No studies available; manufacturers recommend avoidance

Continued

BP
Calcium gluconate

Proprietary

Calcium Gluconate BP (hameln pharmaceuticals Ltd)
Calcium chloride (non-proprietary, see BNF for details)

Group
Electrolytes

Uses/indications
Cardiac resuscitation, acute hypocalcaemia, neonatal tetany
Acute colic of lead poisoning, as an adjunct in the treatment of acute fluoride poisoning and for the prevention of hypocalcaemia in exchange transfusions
NB: calcium gluconate injection is used for the management of magnesium toxicity

Type of drug
POM

Presentation
Sterile injection – each 10-mL ampule, i.e. 950 mg of calcium gluconate, equivalent to 2.2 mmol calcium

Dosage
Cardiac resuscitation: 7–15 mL (1.54–3.3 mmol calcium) under close monitoring including heart rate or ECG (eMC 5/10/2018)
NB: the absolute amount of calcium required for this indication is difficult to determine and may vary widely

Route of admin
IV infusion

Contraindications
Contraindicated in severe renal failure, hypercalcaemia (e.g. in hyperparathyroidism, hypervitaminosis D, neoplastic disease with decalcification of bone), severe hypercalciuria and in patients receiving cardiac glycosides

Side effects

If administered too rapidly, nausea, vomiting, hot flushes, sweating, hypotension and vasomotor collapse which may be fatal

Soft tissue calcification due to extravasation of calcium solutions has been reported

Adverse reactions have been reported in preterm and full-term newborns (aged <28 days) who had been treated with IV ceftriaxone and calcium

Interactions

Digoxin and other cardiac glycosides may be accentuated by calcium, and digitalis intoxication may be precipitated
Increased risk of hypercalcaemia with thiazides

Pharmacodynamic properties

Calcium is an essential body electrolyte
Essential for nerves, and muscle function and contraction, cardiac function and coagulation of the blood

Fetal risks

Should be used only if considered essential

Breastfeeding

Needs to be considered as excreted in breast milk

BP

Naloxone hydrochloride

Proprietary

Naloxone Hydrochloride (ADVANZ Pharma)
Naloxone hydrochloride (non-proprietary, see BNF for details)

Group

Antagonist of central and respiratory depression

Uses/indications

Reversal of postoperative respiratory depression and reversal of neonatal respiratory and CNS depression

Continued

resulting from opioid administration to mother during labour

Type of drug
POM

Presentation
Pre-filled syringe, ampoules

Dosage
Term infant: 200 mcg single dose at birth or in divided doses of 10 mcg/kg every 2–3 min (S.C. or IV) (eMC 8/7/2018)
Preterm infant: smaller dose agreed by paediatrician

Route of admin
IM, IV or S.C.

Contraindications
Hypersensitivity

Side effects
Abrupt reversal of narcotic depression may result in nausea, vomiting, sweating, tachycardia, hyperventilation, increased blood pressure, tremulousness and violent behavior
In postoperative patients, larger than necessary doses of naloxone may result in significant reversal of analgesia and in excitement
Hypotension, hypertension, ventricular tachycardia and fibrillation, hyperventilation and pulmonary oedema have been associated with the postoperative use of naloxone
Seizures have occurred on rare occasions
NB: avoid use in neonates of opioid-dependent mothers as it can precipitate withdrawal symptoms and seizures

Interactions
Unless the stability of naloxone has been established, no drug or chemical agent should be added

Pharmacodynamic properties

An opioid antagonist that is devoid of the morphine-like properties of other antagonists. It acts within 2 min of IV administration but takes longer with IM or S.C. administration, although its effects via these routes last longer

Fetal risk

Crosses the placental barrier but no studies available on its use in pregnancy. Use only if needed

Breastfeeding

Use with caution

NB: Atropine is no longer recommended in the treatment of asystole or pulseless electrical activity.

Drugs Used in the Treatment of Anaphylaxis

Anaphylaxis is a severe, life-threatening, generalized or systemic hypersensitivity reaction. It is characterized by the rapid onset of respiratory and/or circulatory problems and is usually associated with skin and mucosal changes; prompt treatment is required. In addition to the drugs listed below, the following is essential in the treatment of anaphylactic shock.

Oxygen

Oxygen is prescribed for hypoxaemic patients to increase alveolar oxygen tension and decrease the effort of breathing. Oxygen concentration depends on the condition being treated; the administration of an inappropriate concentration of oxygen can have serious or even fatal consequences.

Immediate initiation of high concentration oxygen therapy is required (usually more than 10 L/min) using a mask with an oxygen reservoir. Ensure high-flow oxygen to prevent collapse of the reservoir during inspiration. If the patient's trachea is intubated, ventilate the lungs with high-concentration oxygen using a self-inflating bag.

Intravenous fluids

Large volumes of fluid may leak from the patient's circulation during an anaphylactic reaction. Low blood pressure, vasoconstriction and signs of shock will be evident, so intravenous fluids need to be commenced immediately. There is no evidence to support the use of colloids over crystalloids; therefore, Hartmann's solution or 0.9% saline is suitable.

Bronchodilators

These include inhaled or intravenous **salbutamol**, inhaled **ipratropium**, intravenous **aminophylline** and/or intravenous **magnesium sulphate** (unlicensed).

BP
Adrenaline (epinephrine)

Proprietary
Adrenaline (Epinephrine) Injection 1 : 1000 (Martindate Pharma)

Uses/indications
Anaphylaxis – see Adrenaline under cardiac arrest

BP
Hydrocortisone

Proprietary
Hydrocortisone 100 mg/mL solution for injection (ADVANZ Pharma)
Hydrocortisone 100 mg powder for solution for injection/infusion (Panpharma UK Ltd)
Hydrocortisone sodium succinate (non-proprietary, see BNF for details)

Group
Corticosteroids

Uses/indications
In anaphylaxis (following initial resuscitation) is of secondary value in the initial management of anaphylaxis because the onset of action is delayed for several hours, but should be given to prevent further deterioration in severely affected patients
Suppression of the inflammatory response
Bronchial asthma (see manufacturers' information for other uses)

Type of drug
POM

Presentation
Ampoules – white, freeze-dried powder

Dosage
100–500 mg depending on severity of condition, administered by IV injection over a period of 30 seconds to 1 min
This dose may be repeated 3–4 times in 24 hours as indicated by patient's response and clinical condition (eMC 2/11/2018)

Route of admin
IM, IV

Contraindications
Hypersensitivity to components and in systemic fungal infection, unless specific anti-infective therapy is employed
If live or live-attenuated vaccines are being used in patients receiving immunosuppressive doses of corticosteroids

Side effects
Unlikely as usually only used for short use, but side effects attributable to corticosteroid therapy should be recognized (see manufacturers' information)

Interactions

Drugs that induce hepatic enzymes enhance the metabolism of corticosteroids, so its therapeutic effects may be reduced, e.g. **rifampicin, rifabutin, carbamazepine, phenobarbital, phenytoin, primidone** and **aminoglutethimide**

Convulsions have been reported with concurrent use of **corticosteroids** and **ciclosporin**

Drugs that inhibit the CYP3A4 enzyme, such as **cimetidine, erythromycin, ketoconazole, itraconazole, diltiazem** and **mibefradil**, may decrease the rate of metabolism of corticosteroids and hence increase the serum concentration

Steroids may reduce the effects of anticholinesterases in myasthenia gravis

The desired effects of **hypoglycaemic agents, antihypertensives** and **diuretics** are antagonized by corticosteroids, and the hypokalaemic effects of acetazolamide, loop diuretics, thiazide diuretics and carbenoxolone are enhanced

Efficacy of **coumarin anticoagulants** may be enhanced by concurrent corticosteroid therapy and close monitoring of the INR or prothrombin time is required to avoid spontaneous bleeding

Renal clearance of **salicylates** is increased by corticosteroids, and steroid withdrawal may result in salicylate intoxication

Salicylates and **NSAIDs** should be used cautiously in conjunction with corticosteroids in hypothrombinaemia

Steroids have been reported to interact with neuromuscular blocking agents such as pancuronium, with partial reversal of the neuromuscular block

Pharmacodynamic properties
Anti-inflammatory action
When used in pharmacological doses, its actions
reduce the clinical manifestations of disease in a wide
range of disorders

Fetal risk
The ability of corticosteroids to cross the placenta
varies between individual drugs; however, hydrocortisone readily crosses the placenta which in theory may
result in hypoadrenalism in the neonate, although this
usually resolves spontaneously following birth and is
rarely clinically important

Breastfeeding
Excreted in breast milk, although no data are available
for hydrocortisone

BP
Chlorphenamine maleate

Proprietary
Piriton® (GlaxoSmithKline Consumer Healthcare)
Chlorphenamine injection (Martindale Pharma)
Chlorphenamine maleate (non-proprietary, see BNF
for details)

Group
Antihistamine – sedative

Uses/indications
Emergency treatment of anaphylactic reactions
Adjunctive treatment following adrenaline for ana-
phylaxis
Symptomatic relief of allergy, e.g. hay fever, urticaria

Type of drug
POM

Continued

Presentation
Solution for injection

Dosage
Anaphylactic reaction >12 years and adults: 10 mg
IM or IV slowly (UK Resuscitation Council 2015)
Antihistamine (symptom relief for allergy): see
Chapter 10

Route of admin
S.C., IM, IV
IV route is recommended in anaphylactic reactions
in conjunction with emergency treatment, e.g.
adrenaline (epinephrine), corticosteroids, oxygen and
supportive therapy
Should be injected slowly over a period of 1 min, using the smallest adequate syringe

Contraindications
Hypersensitivity, also in patients who have been
treated with MAOIs within the last 14 days

Side effects
Slight drowsiness to deep sleep, difficulty concentrat-
ing, lassitude, blurred vision, nausea, vomiting and
diarrhoea, urinary retention, headaches, dry mouth,
dizziness, palpitation, painful dyspepsia, anorexia,
hepatitis including jaundice, thickening of bronchial
secretions, haemolytic anaemia and other blood
dyscrasias
Allergic reactions including exfoliative dermatitis,
photosensitivity, skin reactions and urticaria, twitching, muscular weakness and incoordination, tinnitus,
depression, irritability and nightmares
Stinging or burning sensation at the site of
injection
Rapid IV injection may cause transitory hypotension or
CNS stimulation

Interactions

Use with hypnotics/anxiolytics/alcohol may potentiate drowsiness

Inhibits phenytoin metabolism and can lead to phenytoin toxicity

Anticholinergic effects of chlorphenamine are intensified by MAOIs

Pharmacodynamic properties

Acts by competing with histamine for H_1-receptor sites on cells and tissues

Chlorphenamine also has anticholinergic activity

Fetal risk

Use only when the potential benefits outweigh the risks

Use during the third trimester may result in reactions in neonates; for example: irritability, paradoxical excitability, and tremor

Breastfeeding

May inhibit lactation and may be secreted in breast milk

Use only when the potential benefits outweigh the unknown risks

---

BP

Magnesium sulfate heptahydrate (see BNF for details)

Proprietary

Magnesium Sulfate 50% w/v Solution for Injection (Martindale Pharma)

Magnesium sulfate injection (non-proprietary, see BNF for details)

Group

Anticonvulsant – muscle relaxant

Magnesium sulfate is also used (unlicensed) as a tocolytic (see Chapter 20)

Continued

Uses/indications
Pre-eclampsia and eclampsia

Type of drug
POM

Presentation
Ampoules, pre-filled syringe

Dosage
Prevention of seizures in pre-eclampsia
(unlicensed indication): initial IV injection 4 g over
5–15 min, followed by IV infusion, 1 g/h for
24 hours if seizure occurs, additional dose by IV
injection of 2 g (eMC 9/8/2018)
Treatment of seizures and prevention of seizure
recurrence in eclampsia: initially by IV injection 4 g
over 5–15 min, followed by IV infusion, 1 g/h for 24
hours after seizure or delivery, whichever is later; if
seizure recurs, increase the infusion rate to 1.5–2 g/h
or give an additional dose by IV injection of 2 g (eMC
9/8/2018)
NB: for IV injection, concentration of magnesium
sulphate heptahydrate should not exceed 20% (dilute
1 part of magnesium sulphate injection 50% with at
least 1.5 parts of water for injections)

Route of admin
IV injection or infusion

Contraindications
Hepatic and renal impairment, hypersensitivity

Side effects
Hypermagnesaemia, nausea, vomiting, thirst, flushing
of skin, hypotension, arrhythmias, coma, respiratory
depression, drowsiness, confusion, loss of tendon
reflexes, muscle weakness, and following oral administration colic and diarrhea

OVERDOSE: loss of patellar reflexes, weakness, nausea, sensation of warmth, flushing, drowsiness, slurred speech, double vision

NB: according to BNF and manufacturer guidance, ECG monitoring and high-risk observations need to be taken to enable recognition of overdose

Interactions
Caution to patients receiving digitalis glycosides
Magnesium sulphate should **not** be administered together with high doses of **barbiturates**, **opioids** or **hypnotics** due to the risk of respiratory depression
the action of non-depolarizing muscle relaxants such as **tubocurarine** is potentiated and prolonged by parenteral magnesium salts
Profound hypotension if used together with **nifedipine**

Pharmacodynamic properties
Magnesium is involved in neurochemical transmission and muscular excitability, and acts as a depressant on the CNS; peripherally causes vasodilatation
IV administration has an immediate effect that lasts for about 30 min

Fetal risk
Fetal heart rate should be monitored continuously; neurological depression of the neonate includes respiratory depression, muscle weakness and loss of reflexes

Breastfeeding
Secreted but considered safe

Antagonist
Calcium gluconate

BP
Diazemuls

Proprietary

Diazemuls® (Accord-UK Ltd)
Group
Benzodiazepine – sedative, hypnotic, muscle relaxant
Uses/indications
Sedation prior to procedures such as endoscopy, dentistry, cardiac catheterization and cardioversion
Premedication prior to general anaesthesia
Control of acute muscle spasm due to tetanus or poisoning
Control of convulsions, status epilepticus
Management of severe acute anxiety or agitation including delirium tremens

Type of drug
POM

Presentation
Emulsion (made from soya beans)

Dosage

Diazemuls® may be administered by slow IV injection (1 mL/min), or by continuous infusion
Diazemuls® should be drawn into the syringe immediately prior to administration
Sedation: 0.1–0.2 mg diazepam/kg body weight by IV injection (eMC 25/7/2018)
Normal adult dose is 10–20 mg, but dosage should be titrated to patient's response
Premedication: 0.1–0.2 mg diazepam/kg body weight by IV injection (eMC 25/7/2018)
Dosage should be titrated to patient's response

In this indication, prior treatment with diazepam leads to a reduction in fasciculations and postoperative myalgia associated with the use of suxamethonium
Status epilepticus: initial dose 0.15–0.25 mg/kg body weight by IV injection repeated in 30–60 min if required, and followed if necessary by infusion of up to 3 mg/kg body weight over 24 hours (eMC 25/7/2018)
Anxiety and tension, acute muscle spasm, acute states of excitation, delirium tremens: usual dose is 10 mg repeated at intervals of 4 hours, or as required (eMC 25/7/2018) (see manufacturers' guidance for further advice, e.g. continuous infusion)

Route of admin
IM, IV

Contraindications
Hypersensitivity to diazepam, benzodiazepines or any of the excipients, phobic or obsessional states, acute pulmonary insufficiency, myasthenia gravis, sleep apnoea, severe hepatic insufficiency, acute porphyria, use of monotherapy in patients with depression or those with anxiety and depression as suicide may be precipitated, hypersensitivity to egg or soyabean

Side effects
Drowsiness, lightheadedness, confusion, **dependence**; after IV injection there may be a fall in blood pressure and severe respiratory depression; **overdose** (see manufacturers' guidance for detail)

Interactions
Alcohol – enhances sedative effect
Anaesthesia – enhances sedative effect
Antiepileptics – reported both to increase and to decrease plasma phenytoin concentration
Antihistamines – enhanced sedative effect
Antihypertensives – enhanced hypotensive effect

Continued

Pharmacodynamic properties

Diazepam is a potent anxiolytic, anticonvulsant and central muscle relaxant, mediating its effects mainly via the limbic system as well as the postsynaptic spinal reflexes

Fetal risk

Teratogen in the first and second trimesters; prolonged use in the third trimester may cause neonatal respiratory depression, drowsiness, hypotonia and withdrawal

Infants born to mothers who took benzodiazepines chronically during the latter stages of pregnancy may have developed physical dependence and may be at risk of developing withdrawal symptoms in the postnatal period

Breastfeeding

Moderately safe in the short term but avoid repeated doses and observe the infant for lethargy and weight loss

With long-term use, see Fetal risk

References and Recommended Reading

Boyle, M., & Bothamley, J. (2018). *Critical care assessment by Midwives*. London: Routledge.

Briggs, G., Freeman, R., Towers, C., & Forinash, A. (2017). *Drugs in Pregnancy and Lactation: A reference guide to fetal and neonatal risk* (11th ed.). Philadelphia: Wolters Kluwer.

Ciechanowicz, S., & Patil, V. (2012). Lipid emulsion for local anaesthesia systemic toxicity [online]. *Anaesthesiology Research and Practice.* Article ID 131784. Available from: https://www.ncbi.nlm.nih.gov/pmc/articles/PMC3182561/pdf/ARP2012-131784.pdf. [Accessed 28 October 2019].

Croft, J., Draycott, T., Muchatuta, N., & Winter, C. (Eds.). (2017). *PROMPT (Practical Obstetric Multi-Professional Training) Course Manual* (3rd ed.). Cambridge: Cambridge University Press.

Heuser, C., & Branch, D. (2017). Disorders of coagulation in pregnancy. In D. James, P. Steer, C. Weiner, B. Gonik, & S. Robson (Eds.), *High risk pregnancy: Management options* (5th ed.) (pp. 1085–1107). Cambridge: Cambridge University Press.

Intralipid 20% Fat Emulsion 500 mL IV. Baxter Healthcare Ltd. Last updated on the BNF [online] June 2019.

Jordan, S. (2010). *Pharmacology for Midwives: The evidence base for safe practice* (2nd ed.). Basingstoke: Palgrave Macmillan.

Jordan, S., & MacDonald, S. (2017). Pharmacology and the midwife. In S. MacDonald, & G. Johnson G (Eds.), *Mayes' Midwifery: A text book for midwives* (15th ed.) (pp. 158–174). Edinburgh: Elsevier.

Lavonas, E., Drennan, I., Gabrielli, A., Heffner, A., Hoyte, C., Orkin, A., Sawyer, K., & Donnino, M. (2015). Part 10: special circumstances of resuscitation: American Heart Association Guidelines Update for Cardiopulmonary resuscitation and Emergency Cardiovascular Care. *Circulation, 132*(18; Suppl 2), S501–S518. Available from: https://ahajournals.org/doi/full/10.1161/cir.0000000000000264. [Accessed 28 October 2019].

Mavrides, E., Allard, S., Chandraharan, E., Collins, P., Green, L., Hunt, B., et al. (2016). CTG 52 Prevention and management of postpartum haemorrhage [online]. *British Journal of Obstetricians and Gynaecologists, 124*, 106–149. Available from: https://obgyn.onlinelibrary.wiley.com/doi/epdf/10.1111/1471-0528.14178. [Accessed 22 June 2019].

MBRRACE–UK. (2018). *MBRRACE-UK: Saving Lives, Improving Mothers' Care. Lessons learned to inform maternity care from the UK and Ireland. Confidential Enquiries into Maternal Deaths and Morbidity 2014–16.* Oxford: MBRRACE/NPEU. Available from: https://www.npeu.ox.ac.uk/mbrrace-uk/reports. [Accessed 12 April 2019].

National Institute of Health and Care Excellence (NICE). (2010). *CG 107 Hypertension in pregnancy: Diagnosis and management [online].* Last updated January 2011 and checked January 2017. Available from: https://www.nice.org.uk/guidance/cg107. [Accessed 22 June 2019].

National Institute of Health and Care Excellence (NICE). (2011). *CG 132 Caesarean section [online].* Last updated April 2019. London: NICE. Available from: https://www.nice.org.uk/guidance/cg132. [Accessed 22 June 2019].

National Institute of Health and Care Excellence (NICE). (2019). *NG121. Intrapartum care for women with existing medical conditions or obstetric complications and their babies [online].* Last updated April 2019. London: NICE. Available from: https://www.nice.org.uk/guidance/ng121. [Accessed 14 April 2019].

Nursing and Midwifery Council (NMC), 2019. *Standards of proficiency for midwives.* London: NMC. Available from: https://nmc.org.uk/

globalassets/sitedocuments/standards/standards-of-proficiency-for-midwives.pdf. [Accessed 20 November 2019].

Resuscitation Council (UK). (2013). Quality standards for cardiopulmonary resuscitation practice and training: Quality standards and equipment and drug lists for acute care. *Primary Care, Community Hospitals Care [online]*. Last updated May 2017 and March 2018. Available from: https://www.resus.org.uk/quality-standards/. [Accessed 22 June 2019].

Resuscitation Council (UK). (2015). *Resuscitation Guidelines*. Available from: https://www.resus.org.uk/resuscitation-guidelines. [Accessed 18 June 2019].

Royal College of Surgeons (RCS). (2016). *Caring for patients who refuse blood – a guide to good practice for the surgical management of Jehovah's Witnesses and other patients who decline transfusion [online]*. London: RCS. Available from: https://www.rcseng.ac.uk/library-and-publications/rcs-publications/docs/caring-for-patients-who-refuse-blood/. [Accessed 22 June 2019].

Said, S. (2017). Major obstetric haemorrhage and disseminated intravascular coagulation. In D. James, P. Steer, C. Weiner, B. Gonik, & S. Robson (Eds.), *High risk pregnancy: Management options* (5th ed.) (pp. 1986–2014). Cambridge: Cambridge University Press.

Said, S. (2017). Critical care in obstetrics. In D. James, P. Steer, C. Weiner, B. Gonik, & S. Robson (Eds.), *High risk pregnancy: Management options* (5th ed.) (pp. 2015–2067). Cambridge: Cambridge University Press.

SmPC from the eMC. Adenosine 3mg/ml solution for injection. Wockhardt UK Ltd. Last updated on the eMC 15/06/2015.

SmPC from the eMC. Adrenaline 1:1000 injection (glass pre-filled syringe). Martindale Pharma. Last updated on the eMC 20/12/2017.

SmPC from the eMC. Adrenaline 1:10,000 injection (glass pre-filled syringe). Martindale Pharma. Last updated on the eMC 20/04/2018.

SmPC from the eMC. Amiodarone Hydrochloride 50 mg/ml solution for injection or infusion. hameln pharmaceuticals Ltd. Last updated on the eMC 10/01/2019.

SmPC from the eMC. Calcium gluconate injection BP 10 ml ampules. hameln pharmaceuticals Ltd. Last updated on the eMC 05/10/2018.

SmPC from the eMC. Chlorphenamine 10mg/ml solution for injection. Martindale Pharma. Last updated on the eMC 04/01/2019.

SmPC from the eMC. Diazemuls® 5mg/mL emulsion. Accord-UK Ltd. Last updated on the eMC 25/07/2018.

SmPC from the eMC. Hydrocortisone 100mg/ml for injection. AD-VANZ Pharma. Last updated on the eMC 02/11/2018.

SmPC from the eMC. Hydrocortisone 100mg powder for solution for injection or infusion. Panpharma UK Ltd. Last updated on the eMC 01/08/2018.

SmPC from the eMC. Lidocaine 1% solution for injection. Accord Healthcare Ltd. Last updated on the eMC 11/12/2017.

SmPC from the eMC. Magnesium Sulfate 50% solution for injection. Martindale Pharma. Last updated on the eMC 09/08/2018

SmPC from the eMC. Midazolam 1mg/mL, 2mg/mL and 5mg/mL, solution for injection or infusion, hameln pharmaceuticals Ltd. Last updated on the eMC 21/01/2019.

SmPC from the eMC. Narcan® 0.4mg/ml for injection or infusion. AD-VANZ Pharma. Last updated on the eMC 08/07/2018.

SmPC from the eMC. Piriton® 4mg tablets. GlaxoSmithKline Consumer Healthcare. Last updated on the eMC 27/02/2016.

Weiner, C., & Mason, C. (2017). Medication. In D. James, P. Steer, C. Weiner, B. Gonik, & S. Robson (Eds.), *High risk pregnancy: Management options* (5th ed.) (pp. 808–846). Cambridge: Cambridge University Press.

16

Hypoglycaemics

These are agents that reduce the excessive level of glucose in the blood that is a feature of diabetes. Insulin and oral hypoglycaemics play a key role in the regulation of carbohydrate, fat and protein metabolism. Insulin is a polypeptide hormone of complex structure. There are differences in the amino acid sequence of animal insulins, human insulins and the human insulin analogues. Sources of insulin are bovine, porcine or human.

Insulin is a fuel-regulating hormone that controls the amount of glucose in the blood. People with diabetes have a deficiency of insulin and therefore a raised blood glucose level. Four types of insulin are available: fast, short, intermediate and long acting.

Women with insulin-treated diabetes who are planning to become pregnant must be informed that evidence is lacking about the use of long-acting insulin analogues during pregnancy. Therefore, isophane insulin (also known as NPH insulin) remains the first choice for long-acting insulin during pregnancy (NICE 2015, p. 13).

Women with diabetes may be advised to use metformin or glibenclamide as an adjunct or alternative to insulin in the preconception period and during pregnancy, when the likely benefits from improved glycaemic control outweigh potential harm. All other oral hypoglycaemic agents (exenatide and liraglutide) should be discontinued before pregnancy and insulin substituted, as they cross the placenta and may cause severe hypoglycaemia in the neonate.

Hypoglycaemic therapy for women with gestational diabetes may include regular insulin, rapid-acting insulin analogues (aspart and lispro) and/or hypoglycaemic agents (metformin and glibenclamide) should be individualized to each woman.

Women who have been diagnosed with gestational diabetes should discontinue hypoglycaemic treatment immediately after the birth. Women with pre-existing type 2 diabetes who are breastfeeding can resume or continue to take metformin and glibenclamide immediately after birth, but other oral hypoglycaemic agents should be avoided while breastfeeding.

A medical diabetic consultant as well as a consultant obstetrician should care for women who have either insulin-dependent or gestational diabetes. Mixtures of insulin preparations may be required and appropriate combinations have to be determined for the individual patient.

The student should be aware of:

- the physiology and pathology of glucose metabolism
- the treatment of diabetes including emergency management of hypoglycaemic episodes during pregnancy and childbirth
- the methods for diagnosing 'gestational diabetes' and methods of treating the condition
- the modes of insulin administration including insulin pens and insulin pumps for bolus or basal use especially in type 1 diabetes
- the sequelae of pregnancy complicated by diabetes
- local protocols for the care and treatment of mothers with diabetes during antenatal, intrapartum and postpartum periods, and during operative procedures such as LSCS (lower-segment caesarean section)
- care of the neonate after a diabetic pregnancy.

Short-Acting Insulin (Soluble)

- Usually administered 15–30 min before meals
- Effective after 30–45 min
- Peak effect after 1.5–4 hours
- Duration 5–8 hours

Rapid-Acting Insulin

- Before or as soon as possible after meals
- Onset 5–20 min (depending on whether type 1 or 2 diabetes)
- Peak effect after 0.5–0.17 hours (depending on whether type 1 or 2 diabetes)
- Duration 3–5 hours

Intermediate Insulin

- Set times of the day
- Onset 1–2 hours
- Peak effect 6–12 hours
- Duration 12–24 hours

Long-Acting Insulin

- Once daily, at same time
- Onset 2 hours (may vary considerably)
- Peak effect 5–24 hours (no peak)
- Duration 12–24 hours

NB: Human preparations have more rapid onset and shorter durations.

When injected intravenously, soluble insulin has a very short half-life of about only 5 min and its effect disappears within 30 min.

BP
Insulin rapid acting

Proprietary
Apidra® (insulin glulisine) (SANOFI)
Humalog® (insulin lispro) (Eli Lilly and Company Ltd)
NovoRapid® (insulin aspart) (Novo Nordisk Ltd)
Group
Rapid-acting analogue

Uses/indications
Insulin-dependent diabetes mellitus, insulin-dependent gestational diabetes

Type of drug
POM

Presentation
Varied: vial, cartridge, pre-filled pen

Dosage
Dosing is individual and determined in accordance with the needs of the patient

Route of admin
S.C.
Some may be administered by continuous subcutaneous insulin infusion (CSII), intravenously or intramuscularly (see manufacturers' guidance)

Contraindications
Hypersensitivity to the active substance or to any of the excipients

Side effects
Hypoglycaemia, local reactions, fat hypertrophy at injection sites, anaphylaxis
Rarely: peripheral neuropathy
Uncommon: refraction disorders, diabetic retinopathy, lipodystrophy, oedema

Interactions
A number of other medicines may interact with insulin, e.g. oral antidiabetic agents, angiotensin converting enzyme (ACE) inhibitors, fluoxetine, monoamine oxidase inhibitors (MAOIs), salicylates and sulphonamide antibiotics, corticosteroids, diuretics, sympathomimetic agents (e.g. adrenaline (epinephrine), salbutamol, terbutaline), thyroid hormones, oestrogens, progestins (e.g. in oral contraceptives), protease inhibitors and atypical antipsychotic medicinal products (e.g. olanzapine and clozapine) and β-blockers

Continued

Alcohol – enhances the hypoglycaemic effect
Analgesics – salicylates increase insulin requirements
β-blockers – enhance hypoglycaemic effect and mask warning signs, i.e. tremor
Corticosteroids – antagonize the hypoglycaemic effect
Contraceptives – antagonize the hypoglycaemic effect
Nifedipine – may cause impaired glucose tolerance
Smoking – may also antagonize the hypoglycaemic effect of insulin

Pharmacodynamic properties

The primary activity of insulins and insulin analogues is regulation of glucose metabolism

Insulins lower blood glucose levels by stimulating peripheral glucose uptake, especially by skeletal muscle and fat, and by inhibiting hepatic glucose production

Insulin inhibits lipolysis in adipocytes, inhibits proteolysis and enhances protein synthesis

Fetal risk

There are no adequate data on the use of the above in pregnant women

Healthcare professionals should be aware that data from clinical trials and other sources do not suggest that the rapid-acting insulin analogues (aspart and lispro) adversely affect the pregnancy or the health of the fetus or newborn baby (NICE 2015, p. 13)

Breastfeeding

It is not known whether the above rapid-acting insulins are excreted in human milk, but in general insulin does not pass into breast milk and is not absorbed after oral administration

Breastfeeding mothers may require adjustments in insulin dose and diet

BP
Insulin short acting

Proprietary
Actrapid® (Novo Nordisk Ltd)
Humulin S® (Eli Lilly and Company Ltd)
Hypurin Bovine Neutral® (Wockhardt UK Ltd)
Insuman Rapid® (SANOFI)

Group
Short-acting insulin/neutral insulin

Uses/indications
As insulin rapid acting

Type of drug
POM

Presentation
Varied, e.g. vial, cartridge, pre-filled pen, inhaler

Dosage
As insulin rapid acting

Route of admin
S.C.

Contraindications
Hypersensitivity to the active substance or to any of
the excipients hypersensitivity to Humulin or to the
formulation excipients, unless used as part of a desensitization programme
Under no circumstances should any Humulin formulation, other than Humulin S (soluble), be given intrave
nously for hypoglycaemia

Side effects
As insulin rapid acting

Interactions
As insulin rapid acting

Pharmacodynamic properties
As insulin rapid acting

Continued 203

Fetal risk
As insulin rapid acting

Breastfeeding
As insulin rapid acting

BP
Insulin intermediate acting

Proprietary
Humulin I® (intermediate) (Eli Lilly and Company Ltd)
Hypurin® Bovine Isophane (intermediate) (Wockhardt UK Ltd)
Insulatard® (long acting) (Novo Nordisk Ltd)

Group
Medium- and long-acting insulin

Uses/indications
As insulin rapid acting

Type of drug
POM

Presentation
As insulin rapid acting

Dosage
As insulin rapid acting

Route of admin
S.C.

Contraindications
Hypersensitivity to the active substance or to any of the excipients in hypoglycaemia
Cardiac failure has been reported when pioglitazone (oral hypoglycaemic) was used in combination with insulin, especially in patients with risk factors for development of cardiac heart failure
Hypersensitivity to Humulin or to the formulation excipients, unless used as part of a desensitization programme

Under no circumstances should any Humulin formulation, other than Humulin S (soluble), be given intravenously

Side effects
As insulin rapid acting

Interactions
As insulin rapid acting

Pharmacodynamic properties
As insulin rapid acting

Fetal risk
There are no adequate data on the use of the above in pregnant women

Breastfeeding
As insulin rapid acting

BP
Insulin (mixed insulin)

Proprietary
Humulin M3® (Eli Lilly and Company Ltd) – 30% soluble insulin to 70% isophane insulin Insuman Comb 25® (SANOFI) – 25% dissolved insulin and 75% crystalline insulin

Group
Mixed insulin

Uses/indications
As insulin rapid acting

Type of drug
POM

Presentation
Vial, cartridge, pre-filled pen

Continued

Dosage
As insulin rapid acting

Route of admin
Humulin M3® S.C. or IM (not IV), Insuman Comb 25®
S.C.

Contraindications
Hypersensitivity to Humulin or to the formulation
excipients, unless used as part of a desensitization
programme
Under no circumstances should any Humulin formulation, other than Humulin S (soluble), be given
intravenously

Side effects
As insulin rapid acting

Interactions
As insulin rapid acting

Pharmacodynamic properties
As insulin rapid acting

Fetal risk
There are no adequate data on the use of the above
in pregnant women

Breastfeeding
As insulin rapid acting

BP
Insulin long acting

Proprietary
Lantus® insulin glargine (SANOFI)
Levemir® insulin detemir (SANOFI)

Group
Long-acting insulin analogue

Uses/indications
As insulin rapid acting

Type of drug
POM

Presentation
Various: vial, cartridge, pre-filled pen (see manufacturers' guidance)

Dosage
As insulin rapid acting

Route of admin
S.C. (see manufacturers' guidance)

Contraindications
As insulin rapid acting

Side effects
As insulin rapid acting

Interactions
As insulin rapid acting

Pharmacodynamic properties
As insulin rapid acting

Fetal risk
There are no adequate data on the use of the above in pregnant women

Breastfeeding
As insulin rapid acting

BP
Metformin hydrochloride

Proprietary
Metformin hydrochloride (Aurobindo Pharma-Milpharm Ltd)
Metformin hydrochloride (non-proprietary, see BNF for details)

Group
Oral blood glucose-lowering agent

Uses/indications
Type 2 diabetes

Type of drug
POM

Presentation
500 mg film-coated tablets

Dosage
Dosing is individual and determined in accordance with the needs of the patient

Route of admin
Oral

Contraindications
Hypersensitivity, diabetic ketoacidosis, diabetic pre-coma, renal failure or renal dysfunction, severe infection, shock, acute or chronic disease that may cause tissue hypoxia, such as: cardiac failure or recent myocardial infarction, alcoholism/alcohol intoxication, lactation

Side effects
Taste disturbance, nausea, vomiting, diarrhoea, abdominal pain and loss of appetite, erythema, pruritus, urticaria, lactic acidosis, decrease of vitamin B_{12} absorption

Interactions
Alcohol: iodinated contrast agents
Care with glucocorticoids (systemic and local routes), β_2 agonists, and diuretics and ACE inhibitors

Pharmacodynamic properties
Metformin hydrochloride is a biguanide with antihyperglycaemic effects, lowering both basal and postprandial plasma glucose levels
It does not stimulate insulin secretion and therefore does not produce hypoglycaemia

Fetal risk

Manufacturers advise against use in pregnancy; however, NICE (2015) and BNF (2019) indicate strong evidence for its effectiveness and safety in pregnancy

Breastfeeding

Manufacturers advise against use in lactation; however, NICE (2015) and BNF (2019) indicate strong evidence for its effectiveness and safety in pregnancy

References and Recommended Reading

Bailey, J. (2017). Maternal Diabetes Mellitus and Gestational Diabetes. In K. Jackson, & H. Wightman (Eds.), *Normalising Challenging or Complex Childbirth* (pp. 194–214). London: OUP/McGraw Hill Education.

Briggs, G., Freeman, R., Towers, C., & Forinash, A. (2017). *Drugs in Pregnancy and Lactation: a reference guide to fetal and neonatal risk* (11th ed.). Philadelphia: Wolters Kluwer.

Gregory, R., & Todd, D. (2013). Endocrine Disorders. In E. Robson, & J, Waugh (Eds.), *Medical Disorders in Pregnancy: A Manual for Midwives* (2nd ed.). Chichester, West Sussex: Wiley Blackwell.

Jordan, S. (2010). Diabetes mellitus and pregnancy. In S. Jordan (Ed.), *Pharmacology for Midwives: The Evidence Base for Safe Practice* (2nd ed.) (pp. 338–351). Basingstoke: Palgrave Macmillan.

National Institute of Health and Care Excellence (NICE). (2015). *NG3. Diabetes in pregnancy: management from preconception to the postnatal period [online]. Last updated August 2015.* London: NICE. Available from: https://www.nice.org.uk/guidance/ng3. [Accessed 4 April 2019].

National Institute of Health and Care Excellence (NICE). (2019). *NG121. Intrapartum care for women with existing medical conditions or obstetric complications and their babies [online].* London: NICE. Available from: https://www.nice.org.uk/guidance/ng121. [Accessed 14 April 2019].

Nursing and Midwifery Council (NMC). (2019). *Standards of proficiency for midwives.* London: NMC. Available from: https://www.nmc.org.uk/globalassets/sitedocuments/standards/standards-of-proficiency-for-midwives.pdf. [Accessed 20 April 2019].

Rankin, J. (2017). Diabetes mellitus and other metabolic disorders. In J. Rankin (Ed.), *Physiology in childbearing with anatomy and related biosciences* (pp. 361–369). Edinburgh: Elsevier.

SmPC from the eMC. Actrapid® 100iu/mL solution for injection. Novo Nordisk Ltd. Last updated on the eMC 26/03/2018.

SmPC from the eMC. Apidra® 100iu/mL solution for injection. SANOFI. Last updated on the eMC 210/2/2019.

SmPC from the eMC. Humalog® 100iu/mL solution for injection. Eli Lilly and Company Ltd. Last updated on the eMC 29/06/2018.

SmPC from the eMC. Humulin I® (Isophane) 100iu/mL suspension for injection. Eli Lilly and Company Ltd. Last updated on the eMC 29/04/2018.

SmPC from the eMC. Humulin S® (Soluble) 100iu/mL solution for injection. Last updated on the eMC 29/04/2018.

SmPC from the eMC. Humulin M3® (Mixture 3) 100iu/mL suspension for injection in vial. Eli Lilly and Company Ltd. Last updated on the eMC 29/04/2018.

SmPC from the eMC. Hypurin bovine isophane solution for injection. Wockhardt UK Ltd. Last updated on the eMC 04/03/2016.

SmPC from the eMC. Insuman Comb® 25 100iu/mL suspension for injection. SANOFI. Last updated on the eMC 26/04/2019.

SmPC from the eMC. Insulatard® 100iu/mL solution for injection. Novo Nordisk Ltd. Last updated on the eMC 11/05/2018.

SmPC from the eMC. Insuman Rapid® 100iu/mL solution for injection in a cartridge. SANOFI. Last updated on the eMC 29/04/2019.

SmPC from the eMC. Lantus® 100iu/mL solution for injection. SANOFI. Last updated on the eMC 25/02/2019.

SmPC from the eMC. Levemir InnoLet® 100iu/mL solution for injection in pre-filled pen. SANOFI. Last updated on the eMC 25/02/2019.

SmPC from the eMC. Metformin 500mg tablets. Aurobinda Pharma-Milpharm Ltd. Last updated on the eMC 19/03/2019.

SmPC from the eMC. Metformin 500 mg tablets. Wockhardt UK Ltd. Last updated on the eMC 21/06/2017.

SmPC from the eMC. NovoRapid® 100iu/mL solution for injection. Novo Nordisk Ltd. Last updated on the eMC 25/05/2018.

SmPC from the eMC. Tresiba® 100iu/mL cartridge (Penfill). Novo Nordisk Ltd. Last updated on the eMC 21/11/2018.

Wah-Ek Soh, A., Tan, L. K., & Seow-Heong Yeo, G. (2017). Diabetes in Pregnancy. In D. K. James, P. ,J. Steer, C. P. Weiner, B. Gonik, & S. Robson (Eds.) *High Risk Pregnancy: Management Options* (5th ed.) (pp. 1160–1191). Cambridge: Cambridge University Press.

Weiner, C., & Mason, C. (2017). Medication. In D. K. James, P. ,J. Steer, C. P. Weiner, B. Gonik, & S. Robson (Eds.), *High Risk Pregnancy: Management Options* (5th ed.) (pp. 808–840) Cambridge: Cambridge University Press.

Other Resources

Diabetes, U.K., Insulin pens wallchart. Available https://www.diabetes.org.uk/resources-s3/2017-11/insulin-pens-wallchart-autumn-2012.pdf.

See also Diabetes.co.uk

17

Immunoglobulins

These are antibodies, present in the blood, that by specific and direct action defend the body against invading bacteria or organisms. Anti-D immunoglobulin is used prophylactically and in treatment of rhesus iso-immunization in women whose blood is rhesus negative. This immunoglobulin, given via injection, coats fetal cells that may have leaked into the maternal circulation following a sensitizing episode, thus preventing the woman becoming rhesus iso-immunized.

Some antibodies that are present in maternal blood require consultation with the Regional Blood Transfusion Centre as to their relevance to the mother and the fetus/neonate.

Other uses of immunoglobulins include those used as vaccines, i.e. hepatitis, varicella, rubella, tuberculosis, rabies and tetanus, some of which are discussed in Chapter 19.

The student should be aware of:

- blood grouping and rhesus evaluation
- the aetiology of Rhesus iso-immunization
- prevention of iso-immunization
- what action should be taken when there is a possibility that iso-immunization could occur, e.g. in antepartum haemorrhage
- counselling to prevent iso-immunization
- the sequelae to mother and fetus/neonate of rhesus iso-immunization
- the British Society for Haematology guidelines (Qureshi et al. 2014) for administration of anti-D in pregnancy

- an awareness of other antibodies presents in blood, e.g. Lewis, Kell, Duffy anti-E and anti-Fy, etc.
- the sequelae of infection by varicella zoster in pregnant mothers and neonates
- the administration of immunoglobulin to ameliorate the effects of such infection
- the RCOG guidelines (2015) for treatment of varicella zoster contacts.

When evaluating serum titres, the date of the last dose of anti-D should be included on the request document as the antibodies persist in circulation and may give a falsely high reading.

BP
Anti-D (Rh) immunoglobulin

Proprietary

D-GAM® Anti-D Rh Immunoglobulin (Bio Products Laboratory Ltd) – available in 250 IU, 500 IU, 1500 IU and 2500 IU vials – doses according to haematologist instructions
Rhophylac® (CSL Behring UK Ltd)

Group
Immunoglobulins – specific

Uses/indications

Prevention of RhD immunization in RhD-negative women:
- pregnancy/delivery of a RhD-positive baby
- abortion/threatened abortion, ectopic pregnancy or hydatidiform mole
- after antepartum haemorrhage (APH), amniocentesis, chorionic biopsy or obstetrical manipulative procedure, e.g. external cephalic version, or abdominal trauma that may cause transplacental haemorrhage (TPH)

Continued

- treatment of RhD-negative patients after transfusion of RhD-positive blood or other products containing RhD-positive red blood cells (e.g. platelets)
- Rhophylac® (CSL Behring UK Ltd) – see BNF and SPC for detail

Type of drug

POM, Midwives' Exemptions

Presentation

Solution for injection

Dosage

Postnatal dosage: the recommended dose is 500 IU as soon as possible within 72 hours of delivery (additional doses of anti-D should be considered if a large fetomaternal haemorrhage (FMH) is suspected)

Antenatal prophylaxis: 500 IU given at both 28 and 34 weeks of gestation, or a single dose of 1500 IU at 28 weeks' gestation (eMC 6/10/2016)

Following a potentially sensitizing event during pregnancy: administered as soon as possible and no later than 72 hours after the event

- up to 20 weeks' gestation: recommended dose is 250 IU per incident
- after 20 weeks' gestation: recommended dose is 500 IU per incident (a test for the size of the FMH should be performed when anti-D is given after 20 weeks and additional doses of anti-D should be administered as indicated) (eMC 6/10/2016)

Prevention of immunization in RhD-negative patients given blood components containing RhD-positive cells: recommended doses 125 IU/mL of transfused RhD-positive red cells (eMC 6/10/2016)

Students and midwives should consult the NICE Clinical Guidelines (CG37)

Route of admin
D-GAM®, Human Anti-D Immunoglobulin deep IM, S.C. in haemorrhagic disease; also, if more than 5 mL volume doses should be divided and administered at different injection sites

Contraindications
Caution in those who have had an adverse reaction to blood transfusion or to administration of blood derivatives

Hypersensitivity
IM route is contraindicated in persons with severe thrombocytopenia or other disorders of haemostasis

Side effects
Soreness at injection site
Occasionally fever, malaise, headache and chills

Interactions
Live vaccines – if anti-D is given within 2-4 weeks of live vaccine then its action may be impaired

Pharmacodynamic properties
During a sensitizing episode when fetal cells enter the maternal circulation, if they are RhD positive then the body treats them as foreign and makes antibodies against them; this is iso-immunization

When the mother comes into contact with RhD-positive cells again, either later in the same pregnancy or in subsequent pregnancies, her immune system produces immunoglobulins that cross the placenta and destroy fetal blood cells, causing haemolytic disease in the fetus

Anti-D coats fetal cells and disguises them from the maternal immune system so that either the mother remains non-immunized or her system is 'blind' to the fetal cells until they degrade naturally

Fetal risk
N/A

Breastfeeding
No data available

BP
Varicella-zoster virus (live)

Proprietary
Varilrix® (live varicella-zoster virus) (GlaxoSmithKline UK)

Group
Immunoglobulins – specific

Uses/indications
Indicated for active immunization against varicella in healthy adults and adolescents (≥13 years) who are seronegative and at risk

Not indicated for routine use in children, it may be administered to seronegative healthy children 1–12 years of age who are close contacts (e.g. household) of persons considered to be at high risk of severe varicella infections

Type of drug
POM

Presentation
Powder and solvent to prepare solution for injection, vials of solution for injection

Dosage
Varilrix® (live vaccine): two doses (each of 0.5 mL reconstituted vaccine) should be given, with an interval between doses of at least 6 weeks but in no circumstances less than 4 weeks (see BNF 2019)

Route of admin
S.C.

Contraindications
Hypersensitivity to neomycin, severe febrile state, those in an immunocompromised state, pregnancy and breastfeeding

Side effects
Acquiring chickenpox, headache, dizziness, nausea, muscle aches

Interactions
In individuals who have received immune globulins or a blood transfusion, vaccination should be delayed for at least 3 months

Care in children under 16 receiving aspirin and systemic salicylates because of the risk of Reye's syndrome

If a measles-containing vaccine is not given at the same time as Varilrix®, an interval of at least 1 month is recommended between administrations

If another live vaccine is given at the same time, separate injections at different body sites are essential

Pharmacodynamic properties
Infection of the subject with varicella zoster induces the humoral and cell-mediated immune response and thus immunity

Fetal risk
Manufacturers recommend that Varilrix® should not be given to pregnant women as this may cause the fetus to contract chickenpox, to be born with a (mild) form of chickenpox or scars from lesions

May cause respiratory tract problems

Breastfeeding
Women should not be vaccinated while breastfeeding

BP
Varicella zoster immunoglobulin

Proprietary
Human Varicella-Zoster Immunoglobulin (Bio Products Laboratory Ltd)

Group
Immunoglobulins – specific

Uses/indications
Prophylaxis against VZV infection in at-risk patients exposed to varicella (chickenpox) or herpes zoster:
- pregnant women with negative VZV immune status, especially up to early in the third trimester
- neonates whose mothers develop varicella infection within 7 days before and 7 days after delivery
- neonates whose mothers have no history of varicella and/or a negative immune status
- premature infants <28 weeks of gestation or newborns with low birthweight
- Adults and children with no history of varicella and/or a negative immune status, receiving immunosuppressive therapy including steroids, cytostatic agents, radiotherapy, recent stem cell transplantation, or who have congenital or acquired immune deficiency disorders and are not receiving replacement therapy with immunoglobulin

Type of drug
POM

Presentation
Solution for injection

Dosage
Depending on age

Route of admin
IM

Contraindications
Hypersensitivity to any of the components
Hypersensitivity to human immunoglobulins

Side effects

Hypersensitivity, anaphylactic shock, headache, tachycardia, hypotension, nausea, vomiting, skin reaction, erythema, itching, pruritus, arthralgia, fever, malaise, chill and discomfort at site of injection

Interactions

Immunoglobulin administration may interfere with the development of an immune response to live attenuated virus vaccines, such as rubella, mumps and varicella, for a period of up to 3 months
May result in misleading positive results in serological tests

Pharmacodynamic properties

Human varicella-zoster immunoglobulin contains mainly immunoglobulin G (IgG) with a specifically high content of antibodies against VZV

Fetal risk

Clinical experience with immunoglobulins suggests that no harmful effects on the course of pregnancy, or on the fetus and the neonate, are to be expected

Breastfeeding

No evidence to suggest unsafe

References and Recommended Reading

Berlin, C. (2013). Medications and the breastfeeding mother. In D. Mattison (Ed.), *Clinical pharmacology during pregnancy* (pp. 41–54). Edinburgh: Elsevier.

Briggs, G., Freeman, R., Towers, C., & Forinash, A. (2017). *Drugs in Pregnancy and lactation: A reference guide to fetal and neonatal risk* (11th ed.). Philadelphia: Wolters Kluwer.

Herbert, M. (2013). Impact of pregnancy on maternal pharmacokinetics of medications. In D. Mattison (Ed.), *Clinical pharmacology during pregnancy* (pp. 17–40). Edinburgh: Elsevier.

Jordan, S. (2010). Drugs and the immune system. In S. Jordan (Ed.), *Pharmacology for midwives: The evidence base for safe practice* (2nd ed.). Basingstoke: Palgrave Macmillan.

McBain, R., Crowther, C., & Middleton, P. (2015). Anti-D administration in pregnancy for preventing Rhesus alloimmunisation. *Cochrane Database of Systematic Reviews, 2015*(9), CD000020. Available from: https://www.cochranelibrary.com/cdsr/doi/10.1002/14651858.CD000020.pub3/epdf/abstract. [Accessed 18 June 2019].

National Institute of Health and Care Excellence (NICE). (2006). *CG37. Postnatal care up to 8 weeks after birth [online]*. Last updated: 1 February 2015. London: NICE. Available from: https://www.nice.org.uk/guidance/cg37. [Accessed 14 April 2019].

National Institute for Health and Clinical Excellence (NICE). (2008). *TA156 Routine antenatal anti-D prophylaxis for women who are rhesus D negative [online]*. Last updated March 2015. Available from: https://www.nice.org.uk/guidance/ta156. [Accessed 18 June 2019].

Nursing and Midwifery Council (NMC), 2019. *Standards of proficiency for midwives*. London: NMC. Available from https://www.nmc.org.uk/globalassets/sitedocuments/standards/standards-of-proficiency-for-midwives.pdf . [Accessed 20 November 2019].

Qureshi, H., Massey, E., Kirwan, D., Davies, T., Robson, S., White, J., et al. (2014). BCSH guideline for the use of anti–D immunoglobulin for the prevention of haemolytic disease of the fetus and newborn. *Transfusion Medicine, 24*(1), 8–20. Available from: https://onlinelibrary.wiley.com/doi/full/10.1111/tme.12091. [Accessed 18 June 2019].

Royal College of Obstetricians and Gynaecologists (RCOG). (2015). *GTG 13 Chickenpox in Pregnancy [online]*. London: RCOG. Last updated February 2018. Available from: https://www.rcog.org.uk/globalassets/documents/guidelines/gtg13.pdf. [Accessed 18 June 2019].

SmPC from the eMC. D-GAM® 500iu solution for injection. Bio Products Laboratory Ltd. Last updated on the eMC 05/10/2016.

SmPC from the eMC. Human Varicella-Zoster Immunoglobulin (VZIG). Bio Products Laboratory Ltd. Last updated on the eMC 28/03/2019.

SmPC from the eMC. Rhophylac® 300mcg/2mL (1500iu) in pre-filled syringe. CSL Behring UK Ltd. Last updated on the eMC 23/08/2016.

SmPC from the eMC. Varilrix® (live) 10, 3.3 PFU/0.5mL powder and solvent for solution for injection. GlaxoSmithKline UK Ltd. Last updated on the eMC 12/06/2018.

SmPC from the eMC. Varivax® (live) powder and solvent for suspension for injection. Merck Sharp & Dohme Ltd. Last updated on the eMC 29/11/2018.

Varilrix® vaccine powder and solvent for solution for injection 0.5mL vials. GlaxoSmithKline UK Ltd. Last updated on the BNF November 2019.

Watkins, K., Johnson-Roffey, V., Houghton, J., & Robson, S. (2013). Infectious conditions. In E. Robson, & J. Waugh (Eds.), *Medical disorders in pregnancy: A manual for midwives* (2nd ed.) (pp. 215–240). Chichester, WSussex: Wiley Blackwell.

Weiner, C., & Mason, C. (2017), Medication. In D. James, P. Steer, C. Weiner, B. Gonik, & S. Robson (Eds.), *High risk pregnancy: Management options* (5th ed.) (pp. 808–846). Cambridge: Cambridge University Press.

WHO Reproductive Health Library. (2016). WHO recommendation on antenatal anti-D immunoglobulin prophylaxis. The WHO Reproductive Health Library; Geneva: WHO. Available from: https://extranet.who.int/rhl/topics/preconception-pregnancy-childbirth-and-postpartum-care/antenatal-care/who-recommendation-antenatal-anti-d-immunoglobulin-prophylaxis. [Accessed 18 June 2019].

18

Intravenous Fluids

Solutions of electrolytes and water are given intravenously, to meet normal fluid and electrolyte requirements or to replenish substantial deficits or continuing losses, when the patient is unable to take adequate amounts by mouth, e.g. nauseous, vomiting, haemorrhaging, dehydrated or ketotic.

The causes and severity of the electrolyte imbalance must be assessed from the clinical history and biochemical investigations. Sodium, potassium, chloride, magnesium, phosphate and water depletion can occur singly and in combination with or without disturbances of the acid–base balance. Actions must be taken to ensure that circulatory overload does not occur as a result of intravenous fluid therapy, as overloading will result in pulmonary oedema and breathlessness, which may cause respiratory arrest. Hence a record of all fluids infused is essential.

Plasma volume expanders are used for the treatment of circulatory shock, e.g. massive obstetrical haemorrhage or where there is a sudden acute blood or plasma loss leading to a fall in blood pressure and resulting in blood cells collapsing while trying to redress their balance. They restore vascular volume, stabilizing circulatory haemodynamics and maintaining tissue perfusion.

Drugs should **NOT** be added to infusions of sodium bicarbonate, amino acids, mannitol, blood products or specially prepared fat emulsions, such as those used in neonatal intensive care units for feeding neonates (total parenteral nutrition) via the intravenous route.

Instructions regarding storage and degradation of solutions should be noted, and any deviation either from instructions or within the solution should indicate that the infusion should not be commenced, or, if in progress, should be discontinued.

Additive labels should be used to indicate what has been added to the solution, time, strength and, if relevant, expiry time/date, as well as patient identity and the signature of the practitioners checking the infusion. The practitioner must also be aware of the suitability of the additive to the electrolyte solution and where to refer any enquiries.

NB: All fluids should accurately reflect daily requirements, and close monitoring is required to avoid fluid and electrolyte imbalance.

Intravenous fluids are commonly described as crystalloids and colloids.

Crystalloids

These are solutions with small molecules that flow easily from the bloodstream into the cells and tissues. They contain similar concentrations of osmotically active particles to extracellular fluid, so fluid does not shift between the extracellular and intracellular areas. Crystalloids can be described as:

- Isotonic – with a concentration of dissolved particles equal to that of intracellular fluid. Osmotic pressure is therefore the same inside and outside the cells, so they neither shrink nor swell with fluid movement
- Hypotonic – less concentrated than extracellular fluid, so fluid moves from the bloodstream into the cells, causing cells to swell
- Hypertonic – more highly concentrated than extracellular fluid, so fluid is pulled into the bloodstream from the cells, causing cells to shrink.

Intravenous crystalloid fluids in common use

Sodium chloride 0.9% This isotonic solution provides the most important extracellular ions in near physiological concentrations and is indicated in *sodium depletion,* used in fluid replacement and electrolyte balance, as an intravenous infusion, as a carrier for injections in which the prescribed drug requires reconstitution, or as a 'flush' for intravenous cannulae.

Cautions: impaired renal function, cardiac failure, hypertension, peripheral and pulmonary oedema, toxaemia of pregnancy.

Side effects: administration of large doses may give rise to sodium accumulation, oedema and hyperchloraemic acidosis.

NOTE: The term 'normal saline' should not be used to describe sodium chloride intravenous infusion 0.9%; the term 'physiological saline' is satisfactory, but it is preferable to state the actual composition of the fluid, i.e. sodium chloride intravenous infusion 0.9%.

Glucose solutions These are used mostly to replace water deficit and should not be given alone as they may lead to hyponatraemia and other electrolyte disturbances.

Sodium chloride and glucose These hypertonic solutions are indicated when there is combined *water and sodium depletion.* A 1 : 1 mixture of isotonic sodium chloride and 5% glucose allows some of the water (free of sodium) to enter body cells, which suffer most from dehydration, while the sodium salt with a volume of water determined by the normal plasma Na$^+$ remains extracellular.

Glucose 5% This is used as an isotonic intravenous infusion (IVI) for fluid replacement, dehydration and when there is an insulin infusion for the prevention of diabetic ketoacidosis, i.e. during diabetic labours and to provide energy. **NB:** There are a number of different concentrations, i.e. 2.5% and 4% glucose in sodium chloride.

Cautions: becomes hypotonic when the glucose is metabolized; not to be used in resuscitation as can cause hyperglycaemia; care with cardiac and renal disease; and prolonged use does not provide enough daily calories.

Dextrose saline This hypertonic solution of sodium chloride 0.18% plus glucose 4% is contraindicated in hyperemesis due to an increased risk of Wernicke's encephalopathy. If it is necessary to balance electrolytes then give thiamine first and refer to BNF for dosage.

Side effects: hypertonic glucose injections may have a low pH and may cause venous irritation and thrombophlebitis.

Hartmann's solution (compound sodium lactate solution – may be known as 'Ringers' lactate) This isotonic solution, used as an IVI to replace fluid and restore electrolyte balance, can be utilized instead of isotonic sodium chloride solution during or after surgery, or in the initial management of the injured or wounded; it may reduce the risk of hyperchloraemic acidosis. Often used in obstetrics as a carrier for Syntocinon infusions or for 'preloading' before and during epidural analgesia.

Water for injection This is used to reconstitute drugs prescribed as IVI injection.

Intravenous potassium Potassium directly affects how well the body's cells, nerves and muscles function, hence maintaining its balance is essential.

Care must be taken when administering potassium as it is toxic to the heart and so must be given slowly except in extreme circumstances. Hypokalaemia may result if there is renal impairment. Careful patient monitoring is required. Intravenous pumps should be used to control the rate of administration.

Potassium chloride + glucose This is used in severe electrolyte depletion – exact regimen specified by the prescriber.

Potassium chloride + sodium chloride This is used in severe electrolyte depletion – exact regimen specified by the prescriber.

Where possible, premixed infusion solutions should be used or, alternatively, potassium chloride concentrate, as ampoules containing 1.5 g (K$^+$ 20 mmol) in 10 mL, is **mixed thoroughly** with 500 mL sodium chloride 0.9% intravenous infusion. **NB:** Ensure additive label applied externally to the infusion bag.
Potassium chloride + glucose + sodium chloride This is used in severe electrolyte depletion – exact regimen specified by the prescriber.

Colloids

These are also known as plasma expanders/expanders of the intravascular space. They pull fluid into the bloodstream and are used if the circulatory blood volume does not improve. The main concern with colloids is that they may enter the interstitium, resulting in the osmotic gradient being increased and thereby pulling additional water into the interstitium. Increased risk of endothelial injury and capillary leak are linked to thromboembolism, anaphylaxis and disseminated intravascular coagulation (DIC), conditions that often necessitate colloid therapy.

There are four main colloids: albumin, dextran, starches and gelatin.

Albumin

Albumin is derived from human plasma. It is used to maintain normal oncotic pressure and to act as a carrier of some metabolites. Natural colloid, prepared from whole blood, contains soluble proteins and electrolytes but no clotting factors, blood group antibodies or plasma cholinesterases. Albumin can be given without regard to the recipient's blood type.

Albumin solution (human albumin solution) This is a solution containing protein derived from plasma, serum or normal placenta; at least 95% of the protein is albumin. The solution may be isotonic (containing 3.5–5% protein) or concentrated (containing 15–25% protein).

Indications: usually used after the acute phase of illness, to correct a plasma volume deficit.

Cautions: history of cardiac or circulatory disease.

Contraindications: cardiac failure, severe anaemia.

Side effects: hypersensitivity reactions (including anaphylaxis) with nausea, vomiting, increased salivation, fever, tachycardia, hypotension and chills reported.

Isotonic solutions: human albumin solution 4.5%, human albumin solution 5%, Albunorm® 5%, Octalbin® 5% and Zenalb® 4.5%.

Concentrated solutions (20%): human albumin solution 20%, Albunorm® 20%, Flexbumin® 20%, Octalbin® 20% and Zenalb® 20%.

Dextran

This is derived from glucose: Dextran 70 (BNF non-proprietary), RescueFlow® (Dextran 70 intravenous infusion 6% in sodium chloride intravenous infusion) – however, manufacturers advise avoid in pregnancy.

Gelatin

Gelatin is derived from a bovine source: Gelofusine®, Geloplasma® (manufacturer of Geloplasma recommends avoid at the end of pregnancy), Isoplex 4%® and Volplex 4%®.

Starches

Hydroxyethyl starch (HES or HAES) is derived from amylopectin (a soluble polysaccharide); Tetrastarch Volulyte 6% infusion® and Voluven 10% infusion®

The use of HES solutions has been restricted since 2013, and marketing authorisation suspended across the EU from January 2018. Its use to replace plasma volume linked with acute blood loss is associated with serious adverse effects with limited benefits.

NB: It is not within the remit of this book to discuss blood products but it **MUST** be remembered that blood products are drugs and therefore the normal processes in relation to drug administration must be followed alongside the additional requirements set down in Trust policies and procedures.

Midwives' Exemptions

The following may be given by a midwife according to Human Medicines Regulations (Her Majesty's Stationary Office 2012 and amendments 2014 and 2016), Schedule 17, Part 3:

Gelofusine

Hartmann's Solution

Sodium Chloride 0.9%

References and Recommended Reading

Boyle, M., & Bothamley, J. (2018). *Critical care Assessment by Midwives.* London: Routledge.

Crofts, J., Draycott, T., Muchatuta, N., & Winter, C. (Eds.). (2017). *PRactical Obstetric Multi-Professional Training (PROMPT) Course Manual* (3rd ed.) Cambridge: Cambridge University Press.

Dextran 70 with sodium chloride as RescueFlow®. Pharmanovia. Last updated on the BNF [online] April 2019.

Gelofusine 4% infusion in 500mL Ecobags®. B.Braun Medical Ltd. Last updated on the BNF [online] April 2019.

Her Majesty's Stationary Office, 2012. *The Human Medicines Regulations 2012.* London: HMSO. Available from: http://www.legislation.gov.uk/uksi/2012/1916.pdfs/uksi_20121916_en.pdf [Accessed on 12 April 2019].

Her Majesty's Stationary Office, 2014. *The Human Medicines (Amendment) Regulations 2014.* London: HMSO. Available from: http://www.legislation.gov.uk/uksi/2014/490.pdfs/uksi_20140490_en.pdf [Accessed on 12 April 2019].

Her Majesty's Stationary Office, 2016. *The Human Medicines (Amendment) Regulations 2016.* London: HMSO. Available from: http://www.legislation.gov.uk/uksi/2016/186.pdfs/uksi_20160186_en.pdf [Accessed on 12 April 2019].

Jordan, S. (2010). *Pharmacology for Midwives: The Evidence Base for Safe Practice* (2nd ed.). Basingstoke: Palgrave Macmillan.

Mavrides, E., Allard, S., Chandraharan, E., Collins, P., Green, L., Hunt, B., et al. (2016). GTG 52 Prevention and management of postpartum haemorrhage. RCOG: London. *British Journal of Obstetrics and Gynaecology.* 124, e106–e149. Available from: https://obgyn.onlinelibrary.wiley.com/doi/epdf/10.1111/1471-0528.14178 [Accessed 20 May 2019].

MBRRACE–UK. (2018). *MBRRACE-UK: Saving Lives, Improving Mothers' Care. Lessons learned to inform maternity care from the UK and Ireland. Confidential Enquiries into Maternal Deaths and Morbidity 2014–16.* Oxford: MBRRACE/NPEU. Available from: https://www.npeu.ox.ac.uk/mbrrace-uk/reports. [Accessed 12 April 2019].

Nursing and Midwifery Council (NMC). (2019). *Standards of proficiency for midwives.* London: NMC. Available from: https://www.nmc.org.uk/globalassets/sitedocuments/standards/standards-of-proficiency-for-midwives.pdf. [Accessed 20 November 2019].

Rankin, J. (2017). Fluid, electrolyte and acid-base balance. In J. Rankin, J (Ed.), *Physiology in childbearing with anatomy and related biosciences* (pp. 207–216). Edinburgh: Elsevier.

Roberts, J., & Bratton, S. (1998). Colloid volume expanders: Problems, pitfalls and possibilities. *Drugs, 55*, 621–630.

Royal College of Obstetricians and Gynaecologists (RCOG). (2015). *GTG 47 Blood Transfusion in Obstetrics.* London: RCOG. Available from https://www.rcog.org.uk/globalassets/documents/guidelines/gtg-47.pdf. [Accessed 20 May 2019].

Smith, L. (2017). Choosing between colloids and crystalloids for IV infusion. *Nursing Times, 113*(12), 20–23.

SmPC from the eMC. Compound Sodium Lactate solution for infusion. Baxter Healthcare Ltd. Last updated on the eMC 12/12/2018.

SmPC from the eMC. Glucose 5% intravenous infusion. Baxter Healthcare Ltd. Last updated on the eMC 26/9/2018.

SmPC from the eMC. Isoplex® 4% solution for infusion. Beacon Pharmaceuticals. Last updated on the eMC 3/10/2018.

SmPC from the eMC. Potassium Chloride 0.15 % and Glucose 5% solution for infusion. Baxter Healthcare Ltd. Last updated on the eMC 17/2/2016.

SmPC from the eMC. Potassium Chloride 0.15% and Sodium Chloride 0.9% solution for infusion. Baxter Healthcare Ltd. Last updated on the eMC 27/12/2018.

SmPC from the eMC. Potassium Chloride 0.15 %, Sodium Chloride 0.18 % and Glucose 4%, solution for infusion. Baxter Healthcare Ltd. Last updated on the eMC 6/12/2018.

SmPC from the eMC. Sodium Chloride 0.9% intravenous infusion. Baxter Healthcare Ltd. Last updated on the eMC 24/12/2018.

SmPC from the eMC. Sodium Chloride 0.9% solution for injection. ADVANZ Pharma. Last updated on the eMC 24/9/2014.

SmPC from the eMC. Sodium Chloride 0.18% and Glucose 4 % solution for infusion. Baxter Healthcare Ltd. Last updated on the eMC 14/7/2016.

SmPC from the eMC. Sodium Chloride 0.9 % and Glucose 5% solution for infusion. Baxter Healthcare Ltd. Last updated on the eMC 1/6/2016.

SmPC from the eMC. Volplex® 4% solution for infusion. Beacon Pharmaceuticals. Last updated on the eMC 14/8/2018.

SmPC from the eMC. Water for injections. ADVANZ Pharma. Last updated on the eMC 2/4/2019.

SmPC from the eMC. Zenalb® 4.5 (Human Albumin 4.5% solution). Bio Products Laboratory Ltd. Last updated on the eMC 28/1/2013.

SmPC from the eMC. Zenalb® 20 (Human Albumin 20% solution). Bio Products Laboratory Ltd. Last updated on the eMC 11/2/2013.

Wills, L. (Ed.). (2015). *Fluids & Electrolytes Made Incredibly Easy! (Incredibly Easy! Series)* (6th ed.) Philadelphia: Wolters Kluwer.

Volulyte® 6% Infusion 500 ml Freeflex® bags. Fresenius Kabi Ltd. Last updated on the BNF [online] April 2019.

Voluven® 6% Infusion 500 ml Freeflex® bags. Fresenius Kabi Ltd. Last updated on the BNF [online] April 2019.

19

Miscellaneous

This chapter contains the drugs that are used in midwifery and that do not come under any previous title. Specific pre-existing conditions, e.g. asthma, or pregnancy-related conditions, e.g. obstetrical cholestasis, require pharmaceutical treatments that should be familiar to most midwives in clinical practice.

The student should be aware of:

- the non-pregnant physiology and adaptations during childbearing
- the abnormal pathology of pre-existing medical conditions
- the abnormal pathology of pregnancy-related disorders
- the medical management of these conditions during pregnancy, local protocols, and guidance for medication and monitoring of these conditions during childbearing.

Some medications listed here are complementary/alternative medicines. Only a recognized and registered practitioner in the complementary therapy should prescribe any such preparation, just as with conventional medicine one would seek the advice of a doctor or pharmacist prior to taking a medicine.

The student is urged to examine Standard 18 of the Code (NMC 2015) and responsibilities of the midwife (Tiran 2017) on complementary and alternative therapies. Specific consideration of these sources is vital before considering the use of alternative or complementary therapies in any aspect of practice.

BP
Zidovudine (azidothymidine, sometimes known as
AZT – abbreviation to be used with caution as it is also
used for another drug)

Proprietary
Zidovudine (Aurobindo Pharma-Milpharm Ltd), Retro-
vir® (ViiV Healthcare UK Ltd)

Group
Anti-retroviral

Uses/indications
Management of HIV, possibly in the prevention of
maternofetal HIV transmission.
Combination treatments are generally recommended,
e.g. TDF (Tenofovir) with either 3TC (Lamivudine) or
FTC (Emtricitabine) and EFV (Efavirenz).

Type of drug
POM

Presentation
Capsules (white/white hard gelatin capsule), Retrovir
100 mg/10 mL oral solution, vials of 200 mg in 20 mL
solution (10 mg/mL) concentrate for IV infusion

Dosage
*Prevention of maternofetal transmission (over 14 weeks'
gestation):* oral – 100 mg 5 times a day until labour.
Labour and delivery: IV infusion at 2 mg/kg over 1
hour, then 1 mg/kg/h until the cord is clamped
If LSCS planned, commence the regimen 4 hours prior
to delivery (eMC 4/1/2019)

Route of admin
Oral, IV infusion only if unable to take oral formula-
tions and with associated AIDS disorders

Contraindications

Low haemoglobin or neutrophil counts, haematological toxicity: monitor blood levels

Vitamin B_{12} deficiency

Side effects

Multiple, including gastrointestinal disturbances, headache, rash, fever, anaemia

Interactions

Analgesics – methadone increases the plasma concentration of this drug

Antiepileptics – plasma phenytoin concentrations can increase or decrease; valproate – there is a potential for toxicity as plasma levels are increased

Pharmacodynamic properties

A nucleoside reverse transcriptase inhibitor (or 'nucleoside analogue')

Anti-retroviral agent that acts as a virostatic by disrupting viral DNA to inhibit growth and reduce viral numbers

Combination therapy may use protease inhibitors (e.g. Atazanavir), non-nucleoside reverse transcriptase inhibitors (e.g. EFV) and drugs which inhibit fusion of HIV to a host cell (e.g. Enfuvirtide) and others (BNF [online] June 2019)

Fetal risk

Use only if clearly indicated – possible maternal and fetal anaemia

Breastfeeding

General advice is that women with HIV do not breast feed as HIV infection can be transmitted vertically

BP
Aciclovir (acyclovir)

Proprietary
Zovirax® (GlaxoSmithKlein UK)
Aciclovir (Hospira UK Ltd)
Aciclovir (non-proprietary, see BNF for details)

Group
Antiviral

Uses/indications
Treatment of varicella-zoster in pregnancy, herpes zoster, shingles and cold sores

Type of drug
POM

Presentation
Powder for reconstitution, tablets, cream, cold sore cream, suspension

Dosage
Topical: apply to lesion 4-hrly 5 times a day for 5–10 days – prompt recognition and commencement of treatment is recommended (eMC 15/9/2018)
Herpes simplex: Oral: 200 mg × 5 times a day for 5 days or longer (eMC 25/1/2018)
Varicella-zoster: Oral: 800 mg × 5 times a day for 7 days – maintain adequate hydration with higher doses
Slow IV infusion over 1 h – 5 mg/kg t.d.s.
(eMC 25/1/2018)

Route of admin
IV infusion, oral, topical

Contraindications
Renal impairment

Side effects
Multiple, including rash, gastrointestinal disturbances, on IV infusion – local inflammation

Interactions
Ciclosporin and *tacrolimus* – increased risk of ne-phrotoxicity
Mycophenolate and *probenecid* – increased plasma concentration of aciclovir and metabolites of my-cophenolate

Pharmacodynamic properties
A virostatic that interferes with the DNA reproduction function of the virus, reducing production and inhibiting its growth

Fetal risk
Use only when the benefits outweigh the risks, as the number of exposures to the drug is too limited to assess the long-term prognosis

Breastfeeding
Significant amount secreted into breast milk
Oral: 5-day course – considered safe
IV: insufficient information to allow classification as safe

BP
Thyroxine (levothyroxine sodium)

Proprietary
Eltroxin™ (ADVANZ Pharma)
Thyroxine (non-proprietary, see BNF for details)

Group
Thyroid hormone

Uses/indications
Hypothyroidism

Type of drug
POM

Presentation
Tablets (25 mcg, 50 mcg, 100 mcg)

Continued

Dosage
As indicated by laboratory monitoring and the physician

Route of admin
Oral

Contraindications
Thyrotoxicosis, hypersensitivity and adrenal disorders

Side effects
These usually occur with overdose – tachycardia, palpitations, muscle cramps and other indications of an increased metabolic rate

Interactions
Antidepressants – tricyclics, amitriptyline – the antidepressant response is increased by the concurrent use of thyroxine
Anticoagulants – the effect of warfarin is enhanced
Antiepileptics – phenobarbital and phenytoin accelerate the metabolism of thyroxine; phenytoin levels are increased by thyroxine
Cimetidine – reduces the absorption of thyroxine from the gut
Cholestyramine – the absorption of thyroxine is reduced
Iron – ferrous sulphate – reduced absorption of thyroxine
Hypoglycaemics – monitor insulin requirements because of increased metabolic rate
Oral contraceptives – may increase plasma levels of thyroxine

Pharmacodynamic properties
A naturally occurring hormone that contains iodine and is produced by the thyroid gland – required for growth, development and the nervous system
It also increases the basal metabolic rate and has stimulatory effects on heart and skeletal muscle, liver and kidneys

Fetal risk
Monitor serum levels closely

Breastfeeding
Maternal dosage may interfere with neonatal screening for hypothyroidism

---

BP
Salbutamol

Proprietary
Ventolin™ Accuhaler™ (GlaxoSmithKline Ltd)
Salbutamol (non-proprietary, see BNF for details)

Group
Selective β_2-adrenoceptor agonist – bronchodilator short acting (4–6 hours) bronchodilation with a fast onset (within 5 min) in reversible airways obstruction

Uses/indications
Bronchodilator, immediate relief of asthma
Myometrial relaxant: see Chapter 20

Type of drug
POM

Presentation
Pressurized metered-dose inhaler – Accuhaler™ is a multi-dose dry powder inhalation device

Dosage
100–200 mcg (1–2 puffs); for persistent symptoms up to 4 times daily; prophylaxis of allergen or exercise-induced bronchospasm, 200 mcg (2 puffs) duration of action 3–5 hours (eMC 3/8/2015)
Severe acute asthma: Salbutamol Nebuliser Solution (2.5 mg) is indicated for use in the routine management of chronic bronchospasm unresponsive to conventional therapy and the treatment of acute or severe asthma (eMC 22/11/2016)

Premature labour: see Chapter 20 for regime if used as tocolytic

Route of admin

Inhalation

Contraindications

Placenta praevia, antepartum haemorrhage, pre-eclampsia/eclampsia, threatened miscarriage, hypersensitivity

Side effects

Fine tremor (particularly in the hands), nervous tension, headache, muscle cramps

Palpitation, tachycardia, arrhythmias, peripheral vasodilatation, myocardial ischaemia, hypotension, and collapse

Disturbed sleep and behavioural changes

Paradoxical bronchospasm (occasionally severe)

Urticaria, angio-oedema

High doses associated with hypokalaemia

Interactions

β-blockers, e.g. propranolol

Pharmacodynamic properties

Acts on β_2-adrenoceptors of bronchial muscle, with little or no action on β_1-adrenoceptors of cardiac muscle

Fetal risk

Benefit should outweigh the risks; animal studies indicate toxicity at high doses

Breastfeeding

Likely to be secreted in breast milk, so benefits should outweigh risks

BP

Beclometasone dipropionate

Proprietary

Easyhaler® Beclometasone (Orion Pharma UK Ltd)

Beclometasone (non-proprietary, see BNF for details)

Group
Corticosteroid

Uses/indications
Management of chronic asthma – anti-inflammatory action in the lungs

Type of drug
POM

Presentation
Inhalation powder administered from multidose powder inhaler

Dosage
Maintenance: 200 mcg b.d. (eMC 5/4/2017)
Severe: starting dose may need to increase to 600–800 mcg/day and reduced once stabilized
Total daily dose may be administered as 2, 3 or 4 divided doses (eMC 5/4/2017)

Route of admin
Oral inhalation

Contraindications
Hypersensitivity
NB: special care in clients with active or quiescent pulmonary tuberculosis

Side effects
Candidiasis of the mouth and throat (clients are advised to rinse their mouth after using the inhaler)
Hoarseness/throat irritation, cough

Interactions
None reported

Continued

Pharmacodynamic properties

A pro-drug with weak glucocorticoid receptor binding activity, it is hydrolyzed via esterase enzymes to the active metabolite beclometasone-17-monopropionate (b-17-mp), which has high topical anti-inflammatory activity

NB: clients should be instructed in the correct use of the inhaler, and their technique checked, to ensure that the drug reaches the target areas within the lungs
The inhaler must be used regularly (even when asymptomatic for optimal benefit)

Fetal risk

Corticosteroids given to pregnant animals can cause abnormalities of fetal development including cleft palate and intrauterine growth restriction, hence a possible risk to the fetus
Manufacturer recommends use only if benefits outweigh risk

Breastfeeding

Recommend only if benefits outweigh risk

BP

Loperamide hydrochloride

Proprietary

Imodium® (McNeil Products Ltd)
Loperamide hydrochloride (non-proprietary, see BNF for details)

Group

Antidiarrhoeal

Uses/indications

Acute/chronic diarrhea including the symptomatic treatment of acute diarrhoea or acute episodes of diarrhoea associated with irritable bowel syndrome (IBS) in adults

Type of drug

POM

Presentation
Capsules/caplets, syrup, melts or instants

Dosage
Adjusted according to response: usually 4 mg initially and 2 mg after each loose stool thereafter to max dose of 12 mg in 24 hours (max dose 6 mg in IBS), consider fluid and electrolyte depletion – determine and treat underlying cause of diarrhoea (eMC 9/4/2018)

Route of admin
Oral

Contraindications
Abdominal distension, acute ulcerative colitis

Side effects
Abdominal cramps, urticarial, drowsiness, dizziness

Interactions
No data available

Fetal risk
No reports found linking loperamide with either human or animal toxicity, although not advised during first trimester

Breastfeeding
Small amounts of loperamide may appear in breast milk; therefore not recommended in breastfeeding

---

BP
Dexamethasone sodium phosphate

Proprietary
Dexamethasone 3.3 mg/mL injection (hameln pharmaceuticals Ltd)
Dexamethasone tablets (500 mcg to 4 mg), solution (2 mg/5 mL) and injection (3.3 or 3.8 mg/mL)
Dexamethasone (non-proprietary, see BNF for details)

Continued

Group

Glucocorticoid (steroid – synthetic) – anti-allergic, antitoxic, antishock, antipyretic and immunosuppressive properties

Uses/indications

To promote fetal lung surfactant production under 36 weeks' gestation and where labour is imminent/probable; can also ameliorate the effects of cholestasis of pregnancy

Type of drug

POM

Presentation

Tablets, IM injection – glass ampoules

Dosage

NICE NG 25 (2015): IM 6 mg 12 hours apart for 4 doses (do not repeat after max dose) to reduce risk of RDS from preterm birth between 24 and 34 weeks' gestation; effective from 24 hours to 7 days after second dose

Route of admin

Oral, IM

Contraindications

Avoid in suspected chorioamnionitis, tuberculosis, porphyria

Side effects

Rarely anaphylaxis, hypersensitivity, flushing, puerperal rash, fluid retention with repeated doses

Interactions

Analgesics – increases the risk of gastrointestinal bleeding with aspirin and other NSAIDs
Antibiotics – erythromycin may alter the metabolism of corticosteroids

Anticoagulants – alters the effects of anticoagulants, so monitor blood levels closely

Antidiabetics – antagonizes the hypoglycaemic effects

Antiepileptics – phenobarbital, phenytoin and carbamazepine accelerate the metabolism of corticosteroids

Antihypertensives – antagonizes the antihypertensive effect

Pharmacodynamic properties

A glucocorticoid with complex actions, one of which is to promote the production of lung surfactant

It is used to good effect when premature birth is anticipated and ameliorates the effects of cholestasis during pregnancy by reducing serum oestrogen levels

As premature delivery is an outcome of this condition, it also contributes towards reducing neonatal mortality and morbidity

Fetal risk

Overdose can affect the adrenal development of the fetus and neonate, and may contribute to intrauterine growth restriction (IUGR); however, the benefits vastly outweigh the risks of administration

Breastfeeding

No data available – but considered moderately safe if the benefits outweigh the risks

NB: infants of mothers taking high doses of systemic corticosteroids for prolonged periods may have a degree of adrenal suppression

---

BP

Betamethasone sodium phosphate

Proprietary

Betamethasone (RPH Pharmaceuticals AB)
Betamethasone (non-proprietary, see BNF for details)

Continued

Group
Glucocorticoid (steroid)

Uses/indications
To promote fetal lung surfactant production under 36 weeks' gestation and where labour is imminent/probable

Type of drug
POM

Presentation
IM injection – ampoules

Dosage
NICE NG 25 (2015): IM 12 mg 24 hours apart, i.e. 24 mg in total (once only) to reduce risk of RDS from preterm birth between 24 and 34 weeks' gestation; effective from 24 hours to 7 days after second dose

Route of admin
IM

Contraindications
Avoid in suspected chorioamnionitis, tuberculosis, porphyria

Side effects
Rarely anaphylaxis, hypersensitivity, flushing, puerperal rash, fluid retention with repeated doses

Interactions

Analgesics – increases the risk of gastrointestinal bleed with aspirin and other NSAIDs
Antibiotics – erythromycin may alter the metabolism of corticosteroids
Anticoagulants – alters the effects of anticoagulants, so monitor blood levels closely
Antidiabetics – antagonizes the hypoglycaemic effects
Antiepileptics – phenobarbital, phenytoin and carbamazepine accelerate the metabolism of corticosteroids
Antihypertensives – antagonizes the antihypertensive effect

Pharmacodynamic properties
A glucocorticoid with complex actions, one of which is
to promote the production of lung surfactant
It is used to good effect when premature birth is
anticipated

Fetal risk
Fetal teratogenicity at organogenesis; overdosage
can affect the adrenal development of the fetus and
neonate, and may contribute to IUGR; however, the
benefits vastly outweigh the risks of administration

Breastfeeding
Considered moderately safe as there are no controlled
studies involving breastfeeding women and their
infants

BP
Prednisolone

Proprietary
Prednisolone (Accord-UK Ltd)
Prednisolone (non-proprietary, see BNF for details)

Group
Corticosteroid

Uses/indications
Suppress inflammatory and allergic response, e.g.
asthma, immunosuppressive disorders, rheumatic
disease

Type of drug
POM

Presentation
White or yellow tablets

Continued

Dosage

Lowest effective dose to be advised

Initial: 20–40 mg (80 mg in acute conditions) in divided doses with or after food, in the morning – often reduced within days, and then continued under medical supervision until symptoms reduce (eMC 12/12/2018)

Maintenance: 5–20 mg reducing to 2.5–5 mg daily (BNF 2019)

Route of admin

Oral

Contraindications

Systemic infection, hypersensitivity to ingredients

Side effects

Adrenal suppression. Suppression of the inflammatory response and immune function, thus increases susceptibility to infections (enhanced severity)

Severe psychiatric adverse reactions

Avoid exposure to measles and chickenpox (or herpes zoster) – seek urgent medical advice, but continue medication regimen

Increased monitoring should be given for clients with diabetes, hypothyroid conditions, epilepsy or hypertension

Interactions

Anticoagulants – efficacy of coumarin anticoagulants may be enhanced or reduced

NSAIDs – gastrointestinal bleeding and ulceration, renal clearance of salicylates is increased, steroid withdrawal may result in salicylate intoxication

Antibiotics – lower plasma concentrations and enhance renal clearance

Vaccines – avoid as impaired immune response

Hypoglycaemic agents (including insulin), antihypertensives and diuretics – effects likely to be diminished owing to antagonistic effect

Sympathomimetics, e.g. ritodrine, salbutamol, salmeterol, terbutaline – increased risk of hypokalaemia for high-dose usage

Intrauterine device – potential for failure of contraception

Pharmacodynamic properties
Glucocorticoid with anti-inflammatory and immunosuppressive action

Fetal risk
Crosses the placenta – variable, but 88% of prednisolone inactivated during transport
Animal studies have shown cleft palate, IUGR, brain growth and development anomalies
Benefits should outweigh the risks

Breastfeeding
Excreted in small amounts in breast milk; monitor for signs of adrenal suppression in infant, although benefits of breastfeeding are likely to outweigh this risk

---

BP
Clomifene (clomiphene) citrate

Proprietary
Clomid® (SANOFI)
Clomifene (non-proprietary, see BNF for details)

Group
Anti-oestrogen

Uses/indications
Anovulatory infertility

Type of drug
POM

Presentation
Tablets

Continued

247

Dosage
50 mg/day for 5 days after the onset of menstruation; if no ovulation occurs after the first cycle then 100 mg for 5 days – use for a **maximum** of three cycles and under the supervision of a specialist centre (eMC 3/11/2016)

Route of admin
Oral

Contraindications
Pregnancy, hepatic disease, abnormal uterine bleeding, ovarian cysts except polycystic ovaries
CAUTION – with uterine fibroids

Side effects
Menstrual symptoms, hot flushes, abdominal discomfort, withdraw if there are visual disturbances or ovarian hyperstimulation, hair loss, weight gain, rashes, dizziness, rarely convulsions

Interactions
None stated (eMC 2016)

Pharmacodynamic properties
Non-steroidal agent that stimulates ovulation in a high percentage of appropriately selected clients

Fetal risk
Fetal loss, ectopic pregnancy, risk of multiple pregnancy, multiple effects on fetal development, including neural tube defects and trisomies, reported – although not supported by data from population-based studies and still being investigated – therefore pregnancy should be excluded before the next course is commenced

Breastfeeding
Not known to be excreted in breast milk, but thought to reduce lactation

BP
Witch hazel (*Hamamelis virginiana*)

Proprietary
Distilled Witch Hazel (Boots Company PLC)

Uses/indications
Varicosities, perineal trauma, haemorrhoids, herpes lesions

Type of drug
Herbal remedy

Presentation
Liquid

Dosage
As directed by practitioner

Route of admin
Topical

Contraindications
Broken skin/dermal tissue

Side effects
Occasional hypersensitivity reactions

Fetal risk
Safety not established – not recommended

Breastfeeding
Safety not established – not recommended

BP
Calendula officinalis (Marigold)

Uses/indications
Perineal trauma, sore nipples, cystitis, thrush, herpes

Type of drug
Herbal remedy

Presentation
Ointment

Continued

Dosage
As directed by practitioner

Route of admin
Topical

Breastfeeding
Possible risk of allergy that can cause anaphylaxis – therefore considered moderately safe as there are no studies showing increased adverse effects in breastfeeding infants

---

BP
Peppermint water

Uses/indications
To ease colic/flatulence and abdominal cramps

Type of drug
Herbal remedy, also used in aromatherapy

Presentation
Herbal tea: to treat anaemia and mood swings
Herbal suspension/infusion: as indicated above *Essential oil:* to treat nausea and vomiting

Dosage
As directed by practitioner

Route of admin
Oral, inhaled

BP
Arnica montana (leopard's bane or wolf bane)

Proprietary
Boots Bruise Relief Arnica Cream (Boots Company PLC)
Arnica 30c pillules (Boots Company PLC)

Uses/indications
First-aid remedy in bruising and soreness, e.g. episiotomy or other perineal trauma

Type of drug
Homeopathic remedy

Presentation
Pillules or cream

Dosage
As directed by homeopathic practitioner

Route of admin
Oral, topical

Fetal risk
Avoid unless recommended by specialist practitioner

Breastfeeding
No evidence to suggest unsafe

BP
Ursodeoxycholic acid (UDCA)

Proprietary
Ursodeoxycholic Acid (Glenmark Pharmaceuticals
Europe Ltd)
Urdox® (Wockhardt UK Ltd)
Ursodeoxycholic acid (non-proprietary, see BNF for details)

Group
Acts on biliary composition and flow

Uses/indications
Dissolution of bile acids/gallstones (not more than 15
mm in diameter); reduces itching and ameliorates liver
enzymes; used in treatment of intrahepatic cholestasis
of pregnancy (ICP)

Type of drug
POM

Presentation
Tablets, capsules, suspension

Continued

Dosage
Oral: 8–12 mg/kg daily (20–25 g/kg daily – is considered effective and safe) (eMC 9/2/2018)

Route of admin
Oral

Contraindications
Pregnancy

Side effects
Nausea, vomiting, diarrhoea, pruritus

Interactions
Antacids – these bind to bile acids in the gut and have a detrimental effect on mode of action of UDCA
Cholestyramine – binds to bile acids in the gut and has a detrimental effect on mode of action of UDCA
Oestrogens – oral contraceptives – increased bile cholesterol is released, theoretically increasing the effective dose of UDCA

Pharmacodynamic properties
Complex action, but when given orally UDCA dissolves bile acids in the biliary fluid and disperses them, reducing cholesterol and thus ameliorating the cholestasis

Fetal risk
Teratogenic in animal studies and manufacturers advise avoidance during early pregnancy; however, the benefits may outweigh the risks in ICP

Breastfeeding
Manufacturer advises avoidance, but in the absence of controlled study data it is considered moderately safe when treating ICP

BP
Nicotine

Proprietary
Nicorette® (McNeil Products Ltd)
Nicotinell® (GlaxoSmithKline UK Ltd)
NiQuitin® (Omega Pharma Ltd) – various preparations (tablets, patches, lozenges, chewing gum, inhalator see BNF for details)
Champix® (Pfizer Ltd) – varenicline tartrate
Zyban® (GlaxoSmithKlein UK) – bupropion hydrochloride

Group
Nicotine replacement therapy (NRT)

Uses/indications
Smoking cessation regimes where other interventions have not been successful and health benefits are predicted from behavioural change
Electronic/e-cigarettes OR **vaping/vapes** are seen as a safer alternative to cigarette smoking despite the nicotine level consumed being similar (see "E-cigarettes and vaping: policy, regulation and guidance for current information from Public Health England. Available from: https://www.gov.uk/government/collections/e-cigarettes-and-vaping-policy-regulation-and-guidance)
The dangers of nicotine exposure to fetal development during pregnancy and following birth is documented, but further studies of use of electronic/e-cigarettes/vapes for pregnancy and for pregnancy outcomes are needed

Type of drug
POM, some preparations available on GSL – **not** Zyban® or Champix®

Continued

Presentation
Various – see BNF for detail

Dosage

Under NRT guidance of specialist practitioner with counselling and support available

NB: Contraindicated with pregnancy – neuropsychiatric symptoms from varenicline (C) or bupropion (Z)

General dosage advice: Zyban® 150 mg prolonged release film-coated tablets (eMC 26/3/2018), Champix® 0.5 mg film-coated tablets, Champix® 1 mg film-coated tablets (black triangle) (eMC 21/8/2018)

Route of admin
Oral, inhalation, transdermal

Contraindications

Consider risk/benefit assessment before initiating treatment: cardiac conditions (acute myocardial infarction), stroke, renal disease, phaeochromocytoma, hyperthyroidism, other dependencies

Diabetes mellitus – can affect carbohydrate metabolism, thus blood sugar levels should be monitored more closely than usual

Atopic or eczematous dermatitis (due to localized patch sensitivity) – discontinue use and seek medical advice

Side effects

Smoking cessation (general): could suffer from asthenia, headache, dizziness, sleep disturbance, coughing or influenza-like illness

Also depression, irritability, nervousness, restlessness, mood lability, anxiety, drowsiness, impaired concentration and insomnia which may be related to withdrawal

Other: nausea, headaches, faintness, (nicotine) dizziness, coughing or influenza-like illness

Anaphylactic reactions, sleep disorders including abnormal dreams and insomnia, tremor, palpitations, tachycardia, dyspnoea, pharyngitis, cough, nausea, vomiting, dyspepsia, abdominal pain upper, diarrhoea, dry mouth, constipation, sweating increased, allergic dermatitis, contact dermatitis, photosensitivity, arthralgia, myalgia, application site reactions, chest pain, pain in limb, pain, asthenia, fatigue, malaise

Symptoms of **acute nicotine poisoning** include nausea, salivation, abdominal pain, diarrhoea, sweating, headache, dizziness, disturbed hearing and marked weakness

In extreme cases, these symptoms may be followed by hypotension, rapid or weak or irregular pulse, breathing difficulties, prostration, circulatory collapse and terminal convulsions

Management of overdose: stop therapy immediately and admit to hospital, monitor vital signs and ECG, maintain airway, ventilation and oxygenation

Interactions
May possibly enhance the haemodynamic effects of adenosine

Pharmacodynamic properties
Nicotine, an alkaloid in tobacco products and a naturally occurring autonomic drug, is an agonist at nicotine receptors in the peripheral and CNS and has pronounced CNS and cardiovascular effects

Fetal risk
Safety not established; manufacturers recommend smoking cessation without pharmacotherapy wherever possible

Breastfeeding
Compounds secreted in breast milk; manufacturers recommend that the benefit should outweigh the risk from smoking to either mother or baby

References and Recommended Reading

Aziz, N., & Baker, D. (2017). Cytomegalovirus, herpes simplex virus, adenovirus, coxsackievirus and human papillomavirus in pregnancy. In D. James, P. Steer, C. Weiner, B. Gonik, & S. Robson (Eds.). *High risk pregnancy: Management options* (5th ed.) (pp. 660–695). Cambridge: Cambridge University Press.

Briggs, G., Freeman, R., Towers, C., & Forinash, A. (2017). *Drugs in Pregnancy and Lactation: A reference guide to fetal and neonatal risk* (11th ed.). Philadelphia: Wolters Kluwer.

European Medicines Agency (EMA). (2010). *HMPC Assessment Report on Hamamelis virginiana*. London: Ref: EMA/HMPC/114585/2008. EMA.

Hughes, B., & Watts, D. (2017). Human immunodeficiency virus in pregnancy. In D. James, P. Steer, C. Weiner, B. Gonik, & S. Robson (Eds.). *High risk Pregnancy: Management Options* (5th ed.) (pp. 622–644). Cambridge: Cambridge University Press.

Jarvis, S., & Nelson-Piercy, C. (2017). Thyroid disease in pregnancy. In D. James, P. Steer, C. Weiner, B. Gonik, & S. Robson (Eds.). *High risk pregnancy: Management options* (5th ed.) (pp. 1192–1217). Cambridge: Cambridge University Press.

Jordan, S. (2010). Thyroid disorders in pregnancy. In S. Jordan (Ed.). *Pharmacology for midwives: The evidence base for safe practice* (2nd ed.). Basingstoke: Palgrave Macmillan.

Jordan, S., & MacDonald, S. (2017). Pharmacology and the midwife. In S. MacDonald, & G. Johnson (Eds.). *Mayes' Midwifery: A text book for midwives* (15th ed.) (pp. 158–174). Edinburgh: Elsevier.

Medicines and Healthcare products Regulatory Agency (MHRA). Available from: http://www.mhra.gov.uk/ (for information on Arnica, Calendula and Peppermint Water).

Namazy, J., & Schatz, M. (2013). The management of asthma during pregnancy. In D. Mattison (Ed.). *Clinical pharmacology during pregnancy* (pp. 145–156). Edinburgh: Elsevier.

National Institute of Health and Care Excellence (NICE). (2010). *PH26. Smoking: Stopping in pregnancy and after childbirth* [online]. Last updated September 2015. London, NICE. Available from: https://www.nice.org.uk/guidance/ph26. [Accessed 4 April 2019].

National Institute of Health and Care Excellence (NICE). (2013). *PH48. Smoking: acute, maternity and mental health services* [online]. Last updated March 2017, London, NICE. Available from: https://www.nice.org.uk/guidance/ph48. [Accessed 4 April 2019].

National Institute of Health and Care Excellence (NICE). (2015). *NG25. Preterm labour and birth* [online]. London, NICE. Last updated August 2019. Available from: https://www.nice.org.uk/guidance/ng25. [Accessed 19 November 2019].

National Institute of Health and Care Excellence (NICE). (2018). *NG92 Stop Smoking interventions and services* [online]. London, NICE. Available from: https://www.nice.org.uk/guidance/ng92. [Accessed 19 November 2019].

National Institute of Health and Care Excellence (NICE). (2019). *NG121. Intrapartum care for women with existing medical conditions or obstetric complications and their babies* [online]. London, NICE. Available from: https://www.nice.org.uk/guidance/ng121. [Accessed 14 April 2019].

Nursing and Midwifery Council (NMC). (2015). *The code: professional standards of practice and behaviour for nurses, midwives and nursing associates.* Last updated 2018. London: NMC.

Nursing and Midwifery Council (NMC), 2019. *Standards of proficiency for midwives* London, NMC. Available from: https://www.nmc.org.uk/globalassets/sitedocuments/standards/standards-of-proficiency-for-midwives.pdf. [Accessed 20 November 2019].

Riley, L. (2017). Rubella, measles, mumps, varicella and parvovirus in pregnancy. In D. James, P. Steer, C. Weiner, B. Gonik, & S. Robson (Eds.), *High risk pregnancy: Management options* (5th ed.) (pp. 645–659). Cambridge: Cambridge University Press.

Royal College of Obstetricians and Gynaecologists (RCOG). (2011). *GTG 43 Obstetric Cholestasis* [online]. London: RCOG. Available from: https://www.rcog.org.uk/globalassets/documents/guidelines/gtg_43.pdf. [Accessed 23 June 2019].

Royal Pharmaceutical Society (RPS). (2019). *Homeopathy* [online]. Available from: https://www.rpharms.com/resources/quick-reference-guides/homeopathy. [Accessed 5 July 2019].

Smith, M., MacKillop, L., (2017). Respiratory disease in pregnancy. In: James, D., Steer, P., Weiner, C., Gonik, B., & Robson, S., [Eds.]. *High risk pregnancy: Management options.* 5th ed. Cambridge, Cambridge University Press. 944–973.

SmPC from the eMC. Aciclovir® 25 mg/mL concentrated solution for infusion. Hospira UK Ltd. Last updated on the eMC 24/02/2017.

SmPC from the eMC. Betamethasone 4mg/mL solution for injection. RPH Pharmaceuticals AB. Last updated on the eMC 05/04/2018.

SmPC from the eMC. Beclometasone 200 mcg/dose inhalation powder in Easyhaler®. Orion Pharma UK Ltd. Last updated on the eMC 05/04/2017.

SmPC from the eMC. Boots bruise relief Arnica cream. Boots Company PLC. Last updated on the eMC 14/12/2017.

SmPC from the eMC. Boots sore skin relief Calendula cream. Boots Company PLC. Last updated on the eMC 13/01/2012.

SmPC from the eMC. Champix® 0.5mg tablets. Pfizer Ltd. Last updated on the eMC 21/08/2018.

SmPC from the eMC. Clomid® 50mg tablets. SANOFI. Last updated on the eMC 03/11/2016.

SmPC from the eMC. Dexamethasone 3.3 mg/mL solution for injection. hamlen pharmaceuticals Ltd. Last updated on the eMC 28/02/2017.

SmPC from the eMC. Distilled Witch Hazel. Boots Company PLC. Last updated on the eMC 24/03/2015.

SmPC from the eMC. Eltroxin® 25 mcg tablets. ADVANZ Pharma. Last updated on the eMC 02/04/2019.

SmPC from the eMC. Imodium® original 2mg capsules. McNeil Products Ltd. Last updated on the eMC 09/04/2018.

SmPC from the eMC. Lamivudine 150mg tablets. Aurobindo Pharma-Milpharm Ltd. Last updated on the eMC 06/09/2018.

SmPC from the eMC. Nicorette® 2mg gum and Cools 2 mg lozenge. McNeil Products Ltd. Last updated on the eMC 02/06/2016.

SmPC from the eMC. Nicorette® 10mg Invisi patch. McNeil Products Ltd. Last updated on the eMC 27/03/2019.

SmPC from the eMC. Nicorette® 15mg inhalator. McNeil Products Ltd. Last updated on the eMC 30/06/2016.

SmPC from the eMC. Peppermint Water 1973. Martindale Pharma. Last updated on the eMC 29/10/2018.

SmPC from the eMC. Prednisolone 1mg, 2.5mg and 5 mg tablets. Accord-UK Ltd. Last updated on the eMC 12/12/2018.

SmPC from the eMC. Retrovir® 100mg capsules. ViiV Healthcare UK Ltd. Last updated on the eMC 14/02/2018.

SmPC from the eMC. Retrovir® 100 mg/10 mL, oral solution. ViiV Healthcare UK Ltd. Last updated on the eMC 24/12/2018.

SmPC from the eMC. Sustiva® 100 mg capsules. Bristol-Myers Squibb Pharmaceuticals Ltd. Last updated on the eMC 12/03/2019.

SmPC from the eMC. Tenofovir disoproxil 245 mg tablets. Accord Healthcare Ltd. Last updated on the eMC 12/03/2019.

SmPC from the eMC. Ventolin™ Accuhaler™. GlaxoSmithKline Consumer Healthcare. Last updated on the eMC 03/08/2015.

SmPC from the eMC. Ventolin™ 2.5mg Nebules®. GlaxoSmithKline Consumer Healthcare. Last updated on the eMC 22/11/2016.

SmPC from the eMC. Ursodeoxycholic Acid 300mg tablets. Wockhardt UK Ltd. Last updated on the eMC 09/02/2018.

SmPC from the eMC. Ursodeoxycholic Acid 250mg capsules. Glenmark Pharmaceuticals Europe Ltd. Last updated on the eMC 19/03/2019.

SmPC from the eMC. Zidovudine 100mg capsules. Aurubindo Pharma-Milpharm Ltd. Last updated on the eMC 04/01/2019.

SmPC from the eMC. Zovirax® 200mg and 800mg tablets. GlaxoSmithKline Consumer Healthcare. Last updated on the eMC 25/01/2018.

SmPC from the eMC. Zovirax® Cold sore cream. GlaxoSmithKline Consumer Healthcare. Last updated on the eMC 15/09/2017.

SmPC from the eMC. Zyban® 150mg tablets. GlaxoSmithKline Consumer Healthcare. Last updated on the eMC 26/03/2018.

Thomson, A., on behalf of the Royal College of Obstetricians and Gynaecologists. (2019). GTG *73 Care of Women Presenting with Suspected Preterm Pre-labour Rupture of Membranes from Weeks of Gestation* [online]. London: RCOG. Available from: https://obgyn.onlinelibrary.wiley.com/doi/10.1111/1471-0528.15803. [Accessed 23 June 2019].

Tiran, D. (2017). *Complementary therapies and natural remedies in pregnancy and birth: responsibilities of midwives.* In S. Macdonald, G. Johnson, & Midwifery Mayes' (Eds.). (15th ed) (pp. 274–287). Edinburgh: Elsevier.

Weiner, C., & Mason, C. (2017). Medication. In D. James, P. Steer, C. Weiner, B. Gonik, & S. Robson (Eds.). *High risk pregnancy: Management options* (5th ed.) (pp. 808–846). Cambridge: Cambridge University Press.

Myometrial Relaxants

These drugs are sympathomimetics and relax uterine muscle, hopefully preventing premature labour. Their main use is to delay delivery until corticosteroid therapy is complete. Some are used as antagonists to oxytocin, which can cause hyperstimulation of the uterus during the induction or augmentation of labour. Their use is indicated between 24 and 34 weeks' gestation in uncomplicated cases. Other terminology used for this group of drugs is tocolytics (Thomson/RCOG 2019).

The student should be aware of:

- what constitutes premature labour
- local protocols for the management of premature labour
- the sequelae of the action of these drugs on the mother and fetus.

BP
Terbutaline

Proprietary
Bricanyl® injection (AstraZeneca UK Ltd)

Group
Myometrial relaxant/bronchodilator

Uses/indications

Selective β_2-adrenergic agonist for the relief of bronchospasm in bronchial asthma and other bronchopulmonary disorders

To arrest labour between 24 and 33 weeks of gestation in patients with no medical or obstetrical contraindication to tocolytic therapy

The main effect of tocolytic therapy is a delay in delivery of up to 48 hours

Type of drug

POM

Presentation

Ampoules, tablets

Dosage

Tablets 5 mg

Injection – 0.5 mg/mL

As per local protocols (eMC 8/12/2017) or the manufacturers' recommendations – use of syringe pump or controlled infusion device essential (eMC 2/5/2017)

Route of admin

IVI, S.C., IM, oral

Contraindications

Pre-existing ischaemic heart disease or with significant risk factors for ischaemic heart disease

Hypersensitivity

Any condition of the mother or fetus in which prolongation of the pregnancy is hazardous, e.g. severe toxaemia, antepartum haemorrhage, intrauterine infection, intrauterine infection, severe pre-eclampsia, abruptio placentae, threatened abortion during first and second trimester, or cord compression

Side effects

Tachycardia tremor, headache, palpitations paradoxical bronchospasm, an increased tendency to bleeding

Continued

in connection with peripheral vasodilatation, caesarean section, nausea, myocardial ischaemia, hypokalaemia, hypersensitivity reactions including angio-oedema, bronchospasm, hypotension and collapse, arrhythmias, e.g. atrial fibrillation, supraventricular tachycardia and extrasystole, symptoms of pulmonary oedema, mouth and throat irritation, sleep disorder and behavioural disturbances, such as agitation and restlessness, hyperactivity, hyperglycaemia, muscle spasms, hyperlactacidemia, urticaria, rash

Interactions
Beta-blocking agents (including eye drops), especially the non-selective ones such as propranolol, may partially or totally inhibit the effect of β stimulants
Therefore Bricanyl® preparations and non-selective β-blockers should not normally be administered concurrently
Use with caution in patients receiving other sympathomimetics
Hypokalaemia may result from β_2-agonist therapy and may be potentiated by concomitant treatment with xanthine derivatives, corticosteroids and diuretics

Pharmacodynamic properties
Selective β_2-adrenergic stimulant that inhibits uterine contractility

Fetal risk
Administer with caution during the first trimester of pregnancy

Breastfeeding
Secreted into breast milk, but any effects on the infant are unlikely at therapeutic doses
Transient hypoglycaemia has been reported in newborn

BP
Salbutamol

Proprietary
Ventolin™ for IV infusion (GlaxoSmithKline Consumer Healthcare)
Salbutamol 4 mg tablets (Accord-UK Ltd)
Salbutamol (non-proprietary, see BNF for details)

Group
Myometrial relaxant/bronchodilator

Uses/indications
Relief of severe bronchospasm
Management of premature labour; to arrest uncomplicated labour between 24 and 33 weeks of gestation in patients with no medical or obstetrical contraindication to tocolytic therapy

Type of drug
POM

Presentation
Ampoules (5 mg/5 mL), tablets (4 mg)

Dosage

Pre-term labour: Syringe pump or controlled infusion device essential during infusion; the maternal pulse rate should be monitored and rate adjusted to avoid excessive heart rate above 140 beats/min
The volume of fluid infused must be minimized to avoid the risk of pulmonary oedema, hence strict fluid balance records must be kept
Uncomplicated premature labour (between 22 and 37 weeks of gestation) (specialist supervision in hospital)
IV regimen: Initially 10 mcg/min, rate increased gradually according to response at 10-min intervals until contractions diminish then increase rate slowly until contractions cease (maximum rate 45 mcg/min),

Continued

maintain rate for 1 hour after contractions have stopped, then gradually reduce by 50% every 6 hours, maximum duration 48 hours (eMC 30/10/2019)
Maintenance once contractions cease: Salbutamol™ tablets 4 mg given 3 or 4 times daily in divided doses (eMC 30/1/2019)

Route of admin
Oral, IM, IV/infusion (in 5% dextrose – can use NaCl with diabetic patients)

Contraindications
Threatened abortion
Hypersensitivity to any of the components
Pre-existing ischaemic heart disease or those with significant risk factors for ischaemic heart disease

Side effects
Hypersensitivity reactions including angio-oedema, urticaria, bronchospasm, hypokalaemia, hypotension, collapse, tremor, headache, hyperactivity, tachycardia, palpitations, myocardial ischaemia, cardiac arrhythmias including atrial fibrillation, supraventricular tachycardia and extrasystole
Particular to the management of pre-term labour with salbutamol solution for infusion
Nausea, vomiting, muscle cramps, peripheral vasodilatation, pulmonary oedema (patients with predisposing factors including multiple pregnancies, fluid overload, maternal infection and pre-eclampsia may have an increased risk of developing pulmonary oedema)
CAUTION: discontinue if signs of pulmonary oedema or myocardial ischaemia develop

Interactions
Ventolin™ solution for IV infusion should not be administered in the same syringe or infusion as other medications

Salbutamol and non-selective β-blocking drugs, such as propranolol, should not generally be prescribed together

Pharmacodynamic properties
A selective β-antagonist that acts upon receptors in the uterus and bronchi, causing them to relax and lessening contractility

Fetal risk
Little evidence; use with care

Breastfeeding
Probably secreted in breast milk; use with care

BP
Nifedipine

Proprietary
Adalat® (Bayer PLC)
Nifedipine (non-proprietary, see BNF for details)

Group
β2 agonists, calcium channel blocker, hypotensive, vasodilator

Uses/indications
Myometrial relaxant, tocolysis (unlicenced use (BNF [online] June 2019) although use is mentioned in NICE guidance, and hypertension

Type of drug
POM

Presentation
Capsules, tablets

Dosage

Tocolysis: 10 mg stat. sublingually, then 10 mg at 15-min intervals for 1 hour or until contractions have ceased, then 60–120 mg/day via slow-release tablets (or as per local protocol) (maintenance dose 20–40 mg q.d.s.), max dosage 160 mg in 24 hours (BNF 2019) Effective in 30–60 min

Hypertension: see Chapter 11

Route of admin

Oral

Contraindications

Contraindicated in pregnancy before week 20, breast-feeding, hypersensitivity, pre-eclampsia, pre-existing hypotension with systolic below 90 mmHg, previous adverse reaction to calcium channel blockers, cardiac disease – congestive cardiac failure, hepatic dysfunction, aortic stenosis, cardiogenic shock, acute angina attack; should not be administered concomitantly with rifampicin

Side effects

Headache, palpitations, flushing, dizziness, oedema, hypotension, nausea and vomiting

CAUTION: stop treatment if ischaemic pain occurs within 30–60 min of administration

Treatment with short-acting nifedipine, i.e. during a crisis, can induce an exaggerated fall in blood pressure and reflex tachycardia, which may cause complications such as cerebrovascular accident/ischaemia or myocardial ischaemia

Rarely: abnormal liver function tests, congestive cardiac failure, transient hypoglycaemia, tachycardia, chest pain, ischaemia (retinal/cerebral), tinnitus, pruritus An increase in perinatal asphyxia, caesarean delivery, prematurity and intrauterine growth restriction,

although unclear whether this is due to underlying hypertension, its treatment, or to a specific drug effect
EXTREME CAUTION when using magnesium sulphate

Interactions

Do not take with grapefruit juice
Antihypertensives – cause severe hypotension and possible heart failure
Cimetidine – potentiates the hypotensive effect as metabolism of nifedipine is inhibited
Phenytoin – concomitant administration can reduce the effect of nifedipine – monitor plasma levels of anticonvulsants
Erythromycin – may potentiate nifedipine effects
Insulin – possible impaired glucose tolerance

Pharmacodynamic properties

A selective calcium channel blocker with mostly vascular effects
It is a specific and potent calcium antagonist which relaxes arterial smooth muscle, causing arteries to widen and reducing the resistance in coronary and peripheral circulation
This reduces blood pressure and decreases the heart's overall workload

Fetal risk

Toxicity in animals, hypertensive effect can reduce placental flow and cause decrease in fetal oxygenation, i.e. *there is the potential for fetal hypoxia in association with maternal hypotension*
Contraindicated in suspected uterine infection, labour in the presence of placenta praevia, severe intrauterine growth restriction, lethal anomalies or fetal death in utero

Breastfeeding

Should be discontinued if nifedipine treatment becomes necessary during the breastfeeding period

Continued

Other medication that may be used include:

Magnesium sulfate (see Chapter 15) as neuroprotection: give a 4-g intravenous bolus of magnesium sulfate over 15 min, followed by an intravenous infusion of 1 g/h until the birth or for 24 hours (whichever is sooner) (NICE NG 25, 2015).

Tractocile 7.5 mg/mL solution for injection (Atosiban acetate) (Ferring Pharmaceuticals Ltd)

References and Recommended Reading

Adalat® 10mg capsules. Bayer PLC. Last updated on the BNF [online] April 2019.

Briggs, G., Freeman, R., Towers, C., & Forinash, A. (2017). *Drugs in Pregnancy and lactation: A reference guide to fetal and neonatal risk* (11th ed.). Philadelphia: Wolters Kluwer.

Cuppett, C., & Caritis, S. (2013). Uterine contraction agents and tocolytics. In D. Mattison (Ed.), *Clinical pharmacology during pregnancy* (pp. 307–330). Edinburgh: Elsevier.

Jordan, S. (2010). Drugs decreasing uterine contractility: tocolytics. In S. Jordan (Ed.), *Pharmacology for midwives: The evidence base for safe practice* (2nd ed.) (pp. 178–195). Basingstoke: Palgrave Macmillan.

Jordan, S., & MacDonald, S. (2017). Pharmacology and the midwife. In S. MacDonald, & G. Johnson (Eds.), *Mayes' Midwifery: A text book for midwives* (15th ed.) (pp. 158–174). Edinburgh: Elsevier.

National Health Service England (NHSE). (2015). *National Maternity Review: Better Births. Improving outcomes of maternity services in England: A five year forward view for maternity care.* [online]. London, NHSE. Available from: https://www.england.nhs.uk/wp-content/uploads/2016/02/national-maternity-review-report.pdf. [Accessed 4 July 2019].

National Institute of Health and Care Excellence (NICE). (2015). *NG25. Preterm labour and birth [online].* Last updated January 2017. London: NICE. Available from: https://www.nice.org.uk/guidance/NG25. [Accessed 14 April 2019].

National Institute of Health and Care Excellence (NICE). (2010). *CG110. Pregnancy and complex social factors: a model for service provision for pregnant women with complex social factors [online].* Last updated August 2018. London: NICE. Available from: https://www.nice.org.uk/guidance/cg110. [Accessed 14 April 2019].

National Institute of Health and Care Excellence (NICE). (2019). *NG121. Intrapartum care for women with existing medical conditions or obstetric complications and their babies [online]*. London: NICE. Available from: https://www.nice.org.uk/guidance/ng121. [Accessed 14 April 2019].

National Institute of Health and Care Excellence (NICE). (2019). *NG124. Specialist neonatal respiratory care for babies born preterm [online]*. London: NICE. Available from: https://www.nice.org.uk/guidance /ng124. [Accessed 14 April 2019].

Nifedipine 10mg capsules. Strides Shasun (UK) Ltd. Last updated on the BNF [online] April 2019.

Nursing and Midwifery Council (NMC), 2019. *Standards of proficiency for midwives*. London: NMC. Available from: https://www.nmc.org.uk/ globalassets/sitedocuments/standards/standards-of-proficiency-for-midwives.pdf . [Accessed 20 November 2019].

Rang, H., Ritter, J., Flower, R., & Henderson, G. (2016). *Rang and Dale's pharmacology* (8th ed.). Edinburgh: Elsevier Churchill Livingstone.

SmPC from the eMC. Bricanyl® 5mg tablets. AstraZeneca UK Limited. Last updated on the eMC 08/12/2017.

SmPC from the eMC. Bricanyl® 0.5 mg/ml solution for injection or infusion. AstraZeneca UK Ltd. Last updated on the eMC 02/05/2017.

SmPC on the eMC. Ventolin™ solution for IV infusion. GlaxoSmithKlein Consumer Healthcare. Last updated on the eMC 30/10/2019.

SmPC from the eMC. Salbutamol 4mg tablets. Accord-UK Ltd. Last updated on the eMC 30/01/2019.

Thomson, A., on behalf of Royal College of Obstetricians and Gynaecologists (RCOG), (2019). *GTG 73. Care of Women Presenting with Suspected Preterm Prelabour Rupture of Membranes from 24+0 Weeks of Gestation* [online]. London: RCOG. Available from: https://www.rcog.org.uk/en/guidelines-research-services/guidelines/gtg73/. [Accessed 19 November 2019].

Weiner, C., & Mason, C. (2017). Medication. In D. James, P. Steer, C. Weiner, B. Gonik, & S. Robson (Eds.), *High risk pregnancy. Management options* (5th ed.) (pp. 808–846). Cambridge: Cambridge University Press.

21

Oxytocics

Oxytocics (uterotonics) are drugs used to stimulate uterine contractions, i.e. for induction of labour, acceleration of labour, in active management of the third stage, to halt postpartum haemorrhage (PPH) and to control bleeding due to incomplete abortion. In the UK, the oxytocics used are prostaglandins, oxytocin, ergometrine, mifepristone and carbetocin (Pabal®).

The student should be aware of:

- the physiology of labour
- reasons for prolonged, incoordinate labour/contractions
- the physical, psychological and chemical factors that could diminish contractions
- reasons to expedite delivery
- research pertaining to managed and physiological third stage of labour
- appropriate emergency action to be taken in the event of Syntocinon overdose
- the local emergency protocol for postpartum haemorrhage
- the sequelae of oxytocin administration in mother and neonate
- local protocols for the induction and augmentation of labour, including contraindications to therapy, e.g. cord prolapse, cephalo-pelvic disproportion, malpresentation, placenta praevia, antepartum haemorrhage, and cautions in predisposition to uterine rupture, multiple pregnancy, grande multiparity, polyhydramnios, previous caesarean section
- the action of oxytocin, ergometrine and Syntometrine®.

BP
Ergometrine maleate

Proprietary
Ergometrine (hameln pharmaceuticals Ltd)
Ergometrine maleate (non-proprietary, see BNF for details)

Group
Oxytocic

Uses/indications
Ergometrine injection is used in the active management of the third stage of labour and in the treatment of postpartum haemorrhage

Type of drug
POM, Midwives' Exemptions

Presentation
Sterile injection

Dosage
500 mcg ergometrine in 1 mL (eMC 8/5/2018)

Route of admin
IM, IV

Contraindications
Not be used during the first or second stages of labour, or administered to patients with hypertension (including that of pre-eclampsia or eclampsia), occlusive vascular disorders, severe cardiac liver or renal failure or sepsis
The product is also contraindicated in patients with a known hypersensitivity to ergometrine
Special care if given to patients with sepsis or Raynaud's disease

Side effects
Headache, dizziness, tinnitus, cardiac arrhythmias, palpitations, bradycardia, chest pain, coronary arteriospasm with very rare reports of myocardial infarction,

Continued

hypertension, vasoconstriction, dyspnoea, pulmonary oedema, nausea, vomiting, abdominal pain and skin rashes

Interactions

The vasoconstrictor effects of ergometrine are enhanced by sympathomimetic agents

Halothane anaesthesia may diminish the effects of ergometrine on the parturient uterus

Pharmacodynamic properties

Causes sustained contractions of the uterus **within 7 min IM and almost immediately IV**

Sustained uterine contractions

Controls uterine haemorrhage

Fetal risk

Ergometrine use is restricted entirely to the third stage of labour, otherwise it is not recommended for use during pregnancy

Breastfeeding

Ergometrine use is restricted entirely to the third stage of labour, otherwise it is not recommended for use during lactation

---

BP

Ergometrine maleate with oxytocin

Proprietary

Syntometrine® (Alliance Pharmaceuticals)

Syntometrine (non-proprietary, see BNF for details)

Group

Oxytocic

Uses/indications

To expedite placental delivery, to control haemorrhage

Type of drug
POM, Midwives' Exemptions

Presentation
Ampoules

Dosage
One ampoule: ergometrine 500 mcg + oxytocin 5 units in 1 mL (eMC 15/1/2019)

Route of admin
IM

Contraindications
Pre-eclampsia, renal impairment, first and second stages of labour, hepatic, cardiac or pulmonary disease, previous adverse reaction

Side effects
Nausea, vomiting, headache, dizziness, tinnitus, chest pain, palpitations, vasoconstriction, myocardial infarction, pulmonary oedema, stroke

Interactions
Halothane anaesthesia may diminish the uterotonic effect of Syntometrine®
May enhance the effects of vasoconstrictors and prostaglandins

Pharmacodynamic properties
Combines the sustained oxytocic action of ergometrine with the rapid action of oxytocin to act on the smooth muscle of the uterus to expedite placental separation and to control bleeding from the site of placentation after delivery
Syntocinon acts in 2–3 min IM; ergometrine acts in 7 min IM or almost immediately IV

Fetal risk
Causes sustained uterine contraction and restriction of placental blood flow, leading to lack of oxygen to the fetus

Continued

If given to the neonate by accident causes serious and possibly fatal multi-organ shutdown

Breastfeeding
Secreted in breast milk but considered moderately safe

BP
Oxytocin

Proprietary
Syntocinon® (Mylan)
Syntocinon (non-proprietary, see BNF for details)

Group
Oxytocic

Uses/indications
Early stages of pregnancy as an adjunctive therapy for the management of incomplete, inevitable or missed abortion
Induction of labour for medical reasons; stimulation of labour in hypotonic uterine inertia; during caesarean section, following delivery of the child; prevention and treatment of postpartum uterine atony and haemorrhage

Type of drug
POM, Midwives' Exemptions (in emergency situations only)

Presentation
Ampoules (5 units, 10 units)

Dosage

Incomplete, inevitable or missed miscarriage:
by slow intravenous injection, 5 units followed if necessary by intravenous infusion, 0.02–0.04 U/min or faster (eMC 13/2/2018)

For induction or acceleration of labour: according to Trust protocols

Prevention of postpartum uterine haemorrhage: usual dose is 5 IU slowly IV after delivery of the placenta (eMC 13/2/2018)

In women given Syntocinon for induction or enhancement of labour, the infusion should be continued at an increased rate during the third stage of labour and for the next few hours thereafter

Treatment of postpartum uterine haemorrhage: 5 IU slowly IV, followed in severe cases by IV infusion of a solution containing 5–40 IU oxytocin in 500 mL of a non-hydrating diluent, run at the rate necessary to control uterine atony (BNF [online] June 2019)

Route of admin
IM, IV infusion or slow IV injection

Contraindications
Not within 6 hours of prostaglandin administration, intact membranes, hypertonic uterine contractions, mechanical obstruction to delivery, fetal distress, where vaginal delivery is inadvisable, oxytocin-resistant uterine inertia, placenta praevia, vasa praevia, placental abruption, cord presentation or prolapse, severe pre-eclampsia, cardiovascular disease, caution in grande multiparity or where there is predisposition to uterine rupture, polyhydramnios, in cases of IUD or meconium-stained liquor – avoid tumultuous labour as it may cause amniotic fluid embolism

Side effects
Uterine spasm, uterine hyperstimulation, antidiuretic causing water intoxication, hypernatraemia, nausea, vomiting, rashes, **anaphylaxis**, placental abruption, amniotic fluid embolism – where possible, exclude this diagnosis prior to start of therapy

Continued

Interactions

Anaesthetics – can potentiate the hypotensive effect and may cause arrhythmias; the oxytocic effect may be reduced

Prostaglandins – uterotonic effect potentiated

Pharmacodynamic properties

Synthetic form of the hormone oxytocin

It exerts a stimulatory effect on uterine smooth muscle, especially at the end of pregnancy, during labour and post delivery, and in the puerperium when receptors in the myometrium are increased

In low doses it causes rhythmic contractions, but in high doses it causes hypertonic, sustained contractions

Fetal risk

Based on the wide use of this drug and knowledge of its chemical structure and pharmacological properties, it is not expected to present a risk of fetal abnormalities when used as indicated

Fetal distress, asphyxia, IUD

Recent literature identified no correlation between oxytocin in labour and neonatal hyperbilirubinaemia (Sanchez-Ramos and Delke 2017)

Breastfeeding

Considered safe in the newborn because it passes into the alimentary tract where it undergoes rapid inactivation

---

BP
Carbetocin

Proprietary
Pabal® (Ferring Pharmaceuticals Ltd)

Group
Oxytocic

Uses/indications

For the prevention of uterine atony following delivery of the infant by caesarean section under epidural or spinal anaesthesia

Type of drug

POM, authorised by PGD and Midwives' Exemptions

Presentation

Clear colourless solution for injection

Dosage

1 mL Pabal® containing 100 mcg carbetocin – administer only by IV injection, under adequate medical supervision in a hospital

Must be administered slowly, over 1 min, only after delivery of the infant by caesarean section

It should be given as soon as possible after delivery, preferably before removal of the placenta (eMC 30/5/2018)

Route of admin

IV

Contraindications

During pregnancy and labour before delivery of the infant, not for the induction of labour, hypersensitivity, hepatic or renal disease, pre-eclampsia, eclampsia, severe cardiovascular disorders and epilepsy

CAUTION: migraine and hyponatraemia

Side effects

Headache, tremor, hypotension, flushing, nausea, abdominal pain, pruritus, feeling of warmth, anaemia, dizziness, chest pain, dyspnoea, metallic taste, vomiting, back pain, chills and pain

Interactions

Specific interaction studies have not been undertaken; however, as carbetocin is closely related in structure to oxytocin, similar interactions cannot be excluded

Continued

Pharmacodynamic properties

Selectively binds to oxytocin receptors in the smooth muscle of the uterus, stimulating rhythmic contractions of the uterus and increasing the frequency of existing contractions which raises the tone of the uterus musculature

Postpartum carbetocin is capable of increasing the rate and force of spontaneous uterine contractions

The onset of uterine contraction following carbetocin is rapid, with a **firm contraction being obtained within 2 min**

Fetal risk

Contraindicated in pregnancy

Breastfeeding

Small amounts secreted in breast milk

References and Recommended Reading

Berlin, C. Medications and the breastfeeding mother. In D. Mattison (Ed.), *Clinical pharmacology during pregnancy* (pp. 41–54). Edinburgh: Elsevier.

Briggs, G., Freeman, R., Towers, C., & Forinash, A. (2017). *Drugs in Pregnancy and lactation: A reference guide to fetal and neonatal risk* (11th ed.). Philadelphia: Wolters Kluwer.

Cuppett, C., & Caritis, S. (2013). Uterine contraction agents and tocolytics. In D. Mattison (Ed.), *Clinical pharmacology during pregnancy* (pp. 307–330). Edinburgh: Elsevier.

Herbert, M. (2013). Impact of pregnancy on maternal pharmacokinetics of medications. In D. Mattison (Ed.), *Clinical pharmacology during pregnancy* (pp. 17–40). Edinburgh: Elsevier.

Howie, L., & Watson, J. (2017). The third stage of labour. In J. Rankin (Ed.), *Physiology in childbearing with anatomy and related biosciences* (pp. 421–426). Edinburgh: Elsevier.

Jordan, S. (2010). Drugs increasing uterine contractility: Uterotonics (oxytocics). In S. Jordan (Ed.), *Pharmacology for midwives: The evidence base for safe practice* (2nd ed.) (pp. 148–177). Basingstoke: Palgrave Macmillan.

Jordan, S., & MacDonald, S. (2017). Pharmacology and the midwife. In S. MacDonald, & G. Johnson (Eds.), *Mayes' Midwifery: A text book for midwives* (15th ed.) (pp. 158–174). Edinburgh: Elsevier.

MBRRACE–UK, (2018). MBRRACE-UK: Saving Lives, Improving Mothers' Care. Lessons learned to inform maternity care from the UK and Ireland. Confidential Enquiries into Maternal Deaths and Morbidity 2014–16. Oxford: MBRRACE/NPEU. Available from: https://www.npeu.ox.ac.uk/mbrrace-uk/reports [Accessed 12 April 2019].

National Institute of Health and Care Excellence (NICE). (2014). CG190. Intrapartum care for healthy women and babies [online]. Last updated: 21 February 2017. London, NICE. Available from: https://www.nice.org.uk/guidance/cg190 [Accessed 14 April 2019].

National Institute of Health and Care Excellence (NICE), (2019). *NG121. Intrapartum care for women with existing medical conditions or obstetric complications and their babies* [online]. London, NICE. Available from: https://www.nice.org.uk/guidance/ng121 [Accessed 14 April 2019].

Nursing and Midwifery Council (NMC), 2019. *Standards of proficiency for midwives*. London, NMC. Available from: https://www.nmc.org.uk/globalassets/sitedocuments/standards/standards-of-proficiency-for-midwives.pdf [Accessed 20 November 2019].

Sanchez-Ramos, L., & Delke, I. (2017). Induction of labour and termination of pre viable pregnancy. In D. James, P. Steer, C. Weiner, & B. Gonik (Eds.), *High risk pregnancy: Management options* (5th ed.) (pp. 1709–1749). London: Elsevier Saunders.

SmPC from the eMC. Ergometrine 0.05% for injection. hamlen pharmaceuticals Ltd. Last updated on the eMC 08/05/2018.

SmPC from the eMC. Pabal* 100mcg/1mL solution for injection. Ferring Pharmaceuticals Ltd. Last updated on the eMC 30/05/2018.

SmPC from the eMC. Syntometrine* ampoules for injection. Alliance Pharmaceuticals. Last updated on the eMC 15/01/2019.

SmPC from the eMC. Syntocinon* 5iu/mL and 10iu/mL concentrate for solution for infusion. Mylan. Last updated on the eMC 13/12/2018.

Weiner, C., & Mason, C. (2017). Medication. In D. James, P. Steer, C. Weiner, B. Gonik, & S. Robson (Eds.), *High risk pregnancy: Management options* (5th ed.) (pp. 808–846). Cambridge: Cambridge University Press.

Prostaglandins (PGE$_2$)

Prostaglandins are hormones secreted by various body tissues, e.g. uterine and cardiac muscle, semen and the lungs. Prostaglandins are used for cervical ripening and to stimulate the uterus to contract, resulting in labour. Prostaglandins can be administered by a number of routes: vaginal, oral, intravenous, extra-amniotic and intracervical.

Students should be aware of:

■ the indications for induction of labour
■ local protocols for induction of labour – specifically the medication and dosage used
■ the action of prostaglandins with respect to termination of pregnancy and the side effects
■ use of the Bishop's Score in the induction of labour.

BP Dinoprostone	
Proprietary Prostin E$_2$® Vaginal gel and vaginal tablets (Pfizer Ltd) **Group** Prostaglandins **Uses/indications** Induction of labour – cervical ripening for labour when there are no fetal or maternal contraindications	

Type of drug
POM

Presentation
Prostin E_2 Vaginal gel 1 mg, Prostin E_2 Vaginal gel 2 mg, Translucent, thixotropic gel (NICE 2008 does not recommend tablets, IV solution or extra-amniotic solution for induction of labour)
Where tablets are used: Prostin E_2 Vaginal tablets 3 mg

Dosage
CAUTION: Prostin E_2 gel is not a bioequivalent to Prostin E_2 tablets
Dependent on parity, local protocols and Bishop's Score gel should be inserted high into the posterior fornix avoiding administration into the cervical canal
Primigravidas (unfavourable) (Bishop's Score of 4 or less): initial dose of 2 mg administered vaginally
In others: initial dose of 1 mg administered vaginally
In both groups: a second dose of 1 mg or 2 mg may be administered after 6 hours as follows:
- 1 mg should be used where uterine activity is insufficient for satisfactory progress of labour
- 2 mg may be used where response to the initial dose has been minimal
- max dose 4 mg in unfavourable primigravida patients or 3 mg in other patients (eMC 1/2/2018)

The woman should remain left lateral for at least 30 min after administration
Tablet (one) should be inserted high into posterior fornix
A second tablet may be administered after 8 hours
Max 6 mg (eMC 1/2/2018)

Route of admin
P.V. (not intracervical)

Continued

Contraindications

Hypersensitivity, if oxytocic drugs are contraindicated or where prolonged contractions of the uterus are considered inappropriate, e.g. caesarean section or major uterine surgery, potential or obstructed labour, pelvic inflammatory disease (unless adequate prior treatment), active cardiac, pulmonary, renal or hepatic disease

CAUTION: asthma or a history of asthma, epilepsy or a history of epilepsy, glaucoma or raised intraocular pressure, compromised cardiovascular, hepatic, or renal function, hypertension, in women with compromised (scarred) uterus and women aged 35 years or older

Side effects

Asthma, bronchospasm, cardiac arrest, hypertension, rash, diarrhoea, nausea, vomiting, fever, anaphylactoid and anaphylactic reactions including anaphylactic shock, back pain, uterine hypertonus, uterine rupture, abruptio placenta, pulmonary amniotic fluid embolism, rapid cervical dilatation, uterine hypercontractility with/without fetal bradycardia, fetal distress/altered fetal heart rate (FHR), neonatal distress, neonatal death, stillbirth, low Apgar score, warm feeling in vagina, irritation, pain, increased risk of postpartum disseminated intravascular coagulation

Interactions

Oxytocics – uterotonic effect enhanced, hence it is not recommended that these drugs are used together
If used in sequence, uterine activity **MUST** be monitored carefully

Pharmacodynamic properties

A prostaglandin of the E$_2$ series that induces myometrial contractions and promotes cervical ripening

Fetal risk
Abortifacient: exposure to fetal skin in utero causes fetal heart rate abnormalities and may predispose to neonatal jaundice

Breastfeeding
Considered moderately safe, but with extremely limited data on the consequences of administration in breastfeeding women

---

BP
Dinoprostone

Proprietary
Propess® Vaginal delivery system (Ferring Pharmaceuticals Ltd)

Group
Prostaglandins

Uses/indications
Induction of labour – ripening of the cervix for labour when there are no fetal or maternal contraindications

Type of drug
POM

Presentation
A thin, flat semi-opaque polymeric vaginal delivery system which is rectangular in shape with radiused corners contained within a knitted polyester retrieval system

Continued

Dosage

Vaginal delivery system – 10 mg (eMC 16/11/2017)

Administration: Propess® should be removed from the freezer immediately before insertion

The vaginal delivery system should be inserted high into the posterior vaginal fornix using only minimal water-soluble lubricants

Once inserted, the withdrawal tape may be cut, ensuring there is sufficient tape outside the vagina to allow removal

The end of the tape **MUST** not be tucked into the vagina as this would make it difficult to remove

The patient should remain left lateral for 20–30 min after insertion.

Action: Dinoprostone will be released continuously over a period of 24 hours, hence it is important to monitor uterine contractions and fetal condition

If there is insufficient cervical ripening in 24 hours, the vaginal delivery system should be removed

Following the removal of the vaginal delivery system at least 30 min is recommended before oxytocin is commenced

Removal: Gentle traction on the retrieval tape

Removal stops further drug administration when cervical ripening is judged to be complete, e.g. onset of labour, once regular, painful contractions have been established

In multigravidas the vaginal delivery system should be removed irrespective of cervical state to avoid the risk of uterine hyperstimulation, spontaneous rupture of the membranes or amniotomy, uterine hyperstimulation or hypertonic uterine contractions, evidence of fetal distress, maternal systemic adverse dinoprostone effects such as nausea, vomiting, hypotension or tachycardia, at least 30 min prior to starting an intravenous infusion of oxytocin

Route of admin
P.V. (not intracervical)

Contraindications
When labour has started, with other oxytocic drugs, when strong prolonged uterine contractions would be inappropriate, e.g. previous major uterine surgery (caesarean section, myomectomy), cephalopelvic disproportion, fetal malpresentation, fetal distress, more than three full-term deliveries, previous surgery or rupture of the cervix, current pelvic inflammatory disease (unless adequate prior treatment has been instituted), hypersensitivity, placenta praevia or unexplained vaginal bleeding during the current pregnancy

CAUTION: asthma or a history of asthma, epilepsy or a history of epilepsy, glaucoma or raised intraocular pressure, compromised cardiovascular, hepatic or renal function, hypertension, in women with compromised (scarred) uterus and women aged 35 years or older

Side effects
Asthma, bronchospasm, cardiac arrest, hypertension, rash, diarrhoea, nausea, vomiting, fever, anaphylactoid and anaphylactic reactions including anaphylactic shock, back pain, uterine hypertonus, uterine rupture, abruptio placenta, pulmonary amniotic fluid embolism, rapid cervical dilatation, uterine hypercontractility with/without fetal bradycardia, fetal distress/altered FHR, neonatal distress, neonatal death, stillbirths, low Apgar score, warm feeling in vagina, irritation, pain

Interactions
Prostaglandins potentiate the uterotonic effect of oxytocic drugs

Continued

Pharmacodynamic properties

Prostaglandin E_2 (PGE_2) is naturally occurring and found in low concentrations in most body tissues
Cervical ripening involves relaxation of the cervical smooth muscle fibres of the uterine cervix, which must change from a rigid structure to a soft and dilated structure to allow passage of the fetus through the birth canal
Involves activation of the enzyme collagenase, which is responsible for the breakdown of the collagen

Fetal risk

Only used in induction of labour

Breastfeeding

Not indicated for use during lactation

BP

Gemeprost

Proprietary

Cervagem® (SANOFI)

Group

Prostaglandin

Uses/indications

Medical induction of late therapeutic abortion; also used to ripen the cervix before surgical abortion, particularly in primigravidas

Type of drug

POM

Presentation

White to yellowish-white spindle-shaped vaginal pessary

Dosage

Cervagem® 1 mg Pessary (eMC 16/11/2014)
Dependent on stage of pregnancy and indication:
Softening and dilatation of cervix – 1 mg pessary to be inserted into the posterior vaginal fornix 3 hours before surgery
Therapeutic termination of pregnancy – 1 mg pessary to be inserted into the posterior vaginal fornix 3 hourly to a maximum of 5 administrations; a second course of treatment may be instituted starting 24 hours after the initial commencement of treatment
If abortion is not well established after 10 pessaries, a further course of Gemeprost treatment is not recommended and alternative means should be employed to effect uterine emptying
Intrauterine fetal death – 1 mg pessary to be inserted into the posterior vaginal fornix 3 hourly up to a maximum of 5 administrations
The woman should remain left lateral for at least 30 min after administration

Route of admin

P.V.

Contraindications

Hypersensitivity, impaired renal function, chronic obstructive airway disease, cardiovascular insufficiency, raised intraocular pressure, cervicitis, vaginitis; caution with previous uterine surgery or placenta previa, induction of labour or cervical softening at term

Side effects

Vaginal bleeding, mild uterine pain, nausea, vomiting, loose stools/diarrhoea, headache, muscle weakness, dizziness, flushing, chills, backache, dyspnoea, chest pain, palpitations, mild pyrexia, rarely uterine rupture, anaphylactic reactions have not occurred with gemeprost, but such reactions have very rarely been noted with other prostaglandins; severe hypotension and coronary spasms with resulting myocardial infarction has been reported rarely

NB: careful monitoring of blood pressure and pulse essential for 3 hours after administration due to risk of profound hypotension

Interactions
Oxytocics – enhances uterotonic effect

Pharmacodynamic properties
Causes contraction of the uterus and softening which decreases resistance of cervical tissue, depresses placental and uterine blood flow, but these actions are secondary to the main uterine stimulation

Fetal risk
Abortifacient

Breastfeeding
Not applicable

BP
Carboprost tromethamine

Proprietary
Hemabate® Sterile Solution (Pfizer Limited)

Group
Synthetic prostaglandin (F2α) following oxytocin or ergometrine

Uses/indications
Treatment of uterine atony in postpartum haemorrhage when ergometrine and oxytocin have already been used

Type of drug
POM

Presentation
Solution for injection

Dosage
1 mL contains carboprost tromethamine equivalent to carboprost 250 mcg

An initial dose of 250 mcg (1.0 mL) Hemabate as a deep IM injection

If necessary, further doses of 250 mcg may be administered at intervals of approximately 1.5 hours

In severe cases the interval between doses may be reduced but it should not be less than 15 min

The total dose of Hemabate should not exceed 2 mg (8 doses) (eMC 10/10/2013)

Route of admin
Deep IM injection or injection into the lower uterine segment to control severe haemorrhage

Contraindications
Hypersensitivity, acute pelvic inflammatory disease, known active cardiac, pulmonary, renal, or hepatic disease

NB: assessment of the benefit/risk ratio may be necessary

Side effects
Headache, flushing, hot flushes, chills, cough and body temperature increase

Interactions
Enhance the effect of other oxytocics

Pharmacodynamic properties
Stimulates the uterus to contract to promote homeostasis at the placental site and prevents further blood loss

Prostaglandins stimulate the smooth muscle to contract and inhibit the release of noradrenaline (norepinephrine)

Fetal risk
Not applicable

Breastfeeding
No evidence to say unsafe

BP
Mifepristone

Proprietary
Mifegyne® (Exelgyn)

Group
Antiprogestogenic steroid

Uses/indications
Medical termination of developing intrauterine pregnancy

Softening and dilatation of the cervix prior to surgical termination of pregnancy during the first trimester

Preparation for the action of prostaglandin analogues in the termination of pregnancy for medical reasons (*beyond the first trimester*)

Induction for intrauterine death where prostaglandin or oxytocin are contraindicated

Type of drug
POM

Presentation
Light yellow, cylindrical, bi-convex tablets

Dosage
Gestation up to 9 weeks: mifepristone 200 mg orally followed 1–3 days later by misoprostol 800 mcg vaginally; in women at more than 7 weeks' gestation (49–63 days), if the abortion has not occurred 4 hours after misoprostol, a further dose of misoprostol 400 mcg may be given vaginally or orally (eMC 11/8/2017)

Gestation between 9 and 13 weeks: mifepristone 200 mg orally followed 36–48 hours later by misoprostol 800 mcg vaginally followed if necessary by a maximum of 4 further doses at 3 hourly intervals of misoprostol 400 mcg vaginally or orally (eMC 11/8/2017)

Gestation between 13 and 24 weeks: mifepristone 200 mg orally followed 36–48 hours later by misoprostol 800 mcg vaginally, then a maximum of 4 further doses at 3 hourly intervals of misoprostol 400 mcg orally (eMC 11/8/2017)

Route of admin

Oral

Contraindications

SHOULD NEVER be prescribed if: chronic adrenal failure, hypersensitivity, severe asthma (uncontrolled by therapy) or inherited porphyria

See SPC for specific contraindications in relation to the indications for use

Side effects

Headache, nausea, vomiting, diarrhoea, cramping, hypersensitivity: skin rashes, urticaria, erythroderma, erythema nodosum, toxic epidermal necrolysis, infection (endometritis, pelvic inflammatory disease), toxic shock, hypotension, malaise, hot flushes, dizziness, chills, fever, and uterine rupture

Interactions

Mifepristone is a CYP3A4 substrate and metabolized by CYP3A4 (a cytochrome P450 enzyme)

It is likely that ketoconazole, itraconazole, erythromycin and grapefruit juice may inhibit its metabolism (increasing serum levels of mifepristone) and toxicity also in the presence of CYP3A4 inhibitors and inducers

Rifampicin, dexamethasone, St John's wort and certain anticonvulsants (phenytoin, phenobarbital, carbamazepine) may induce mifepristone metabolism (lowering serum levels of mifepristone)

General anaesthetic may also enhance mifepristone toxicity

Continued

Pharmacodynamic properties
During pregnancy it sensitizes the myometrium to the contraction-inducing action of prostaglandin

Fetal risk
Data are too limited to determine teratogenicity, so if the method of termination fails further methods should be tried

NB: if the woman wishes to continue the pregnancy, close ultrasonographic follow-up is recommended

Breastfeeding
No data are available; therefore, should be avoided during breastfeeding

---

BP
Misoprostol

Proprietary
Cytotec® (Pfizer Limited)
Misoprostol (non-proprietary, see BNF for details)

Group
Synthetic prostaglandin

Uses/indications
Currently not licensed to induce medical abortion
Currently not licensed in postpartum haemorrhage
Used when oxytocin, ergometrine and carboprost are not available

Type of drug
Prostaglandin

Presentation
White to off-white hexagonal tablets

Dosage
See **Mifeprostone** in relation to termination of pregnancy
PPH prevention – 600 mg orally (when oxytocic not available) (RCOG GTG 52, 2016)
PPH treatment – 1000 mg rectally (RCOG GTG 52, 2016)

Route of admin
Oral or vaginal

Contraindications
Women who are pregnant, or in whom pregnancy has not been excluded, or women planning a pregnancy as misoprostol increases uterine tone and contractions in pregnancy which may cause partial or complete expulsion of the products of conception
However, used to induce medical abortion (unlicensed) – see BNF for details

Side effects
Anaphylactic reaction, dizziness, headache, diarrhoea, abdominal pain, constipation, dyspepsia, flatulence, nausea, vomiting, rash, amniotic fluid embolism, abnormal uterine contractions, fetal death, incomplete abortion, premature birth, retained placenta, uterine rupture, uterine perforation, vaginal haemorrhage (including postmenopausal bleeding), intermenstrual bleeding, menstrual disorder, uterine cramping, menorrhagia, dysmenorrhoea, uterine haemorrhage, birth defects, chills and pyrexia

Interactions
In rare cases NSAIDs and misoprostol may cause a transaminase increase and peripheral oedema
Drug interaction studies have shown no significance in relation to and several NSAIDs, diclofenac, piroxicam, aspirin, naproxen or indomethacin
Magnesium-containing antacids should be avoided during treatment with misoprostol as this may worsen the misoprostol-induced diarrhoea

Continued

Pharmacodynamic properties

Increases uterine tone and contractions in pregnancy which may cause partial or complete expulsion of the products of conception

An analogue of naturally occurring prostaglandin E_1, which promotes peptic ulcer healing and provides symptomatic relief

Protects the gastroduodenal mucosa by inhibiting basal, stimulated and nocturnal acid secretion, and by reducing the volume of gastric secretions, the proteolytic activity of the gastric fluid, and increasing bicarbonate and mucus secretion

Fetal risk

Associated with abortion, premature birth, and fetal death and birth defects

Breastfeeding

Should not be administered to nursing mothers as causes diarrhoea in infants

References and Recommended Reading

Balchin, I., Breeze, A., & Steer, P. (2017). Prolonged pregnancy. In D. James, P. Steer, C. Weiner, B. Gonik, & S. Robson (Eds.), *High risk pregnancy: Management options* (5th ed.) (pp. 1697–1708). Cambridge: Cambridge University Press.

Howie, L., & Marshall, H. (2017). Abnormalities of uterine action and onset of labour. In J. Rankin (Ed.), *Physiology in childbearing with anatomy and related biosciences* (pp. 429–439). Edinburgh: Elsevier.

Jordan, S. (2010). *Pharmacology for midwives: The evidence base for safe practice* (2nd ed.). Basingstoke: Palgrave Macmillan.

Mavrides, E., Allard, S., Chandraharan, E., Collins, P., Green, L., Hunt, B., et al. (2016). *GTG 52 Postpartum Haemorrhage, Prevention and Management* [online]. London, RCOG. Available from: https://obgyn.onlinelibrary.wiley.com/doi/epdf/10.1111/1471-0528.14178. [Accessed 23 June 2019].

MBRRACE–UK. (2018). MBRRACE-UK: Saving Lives, Improving Mothers' Care. Lessons learned to inform maternity care from the UK and Ireland. Confidential Enquiries into Maternal Deaths and Morbidity 2014–16. Oxford: MBRRACE/NPEU. Available from: https://www.npeu.ox.ac.uk/mbrrace-uk/reports. [Accessed 12 April 2019]

National Institute of Health and Care Excellence (NICE), (2008). *CG70. Inducing labour* [online]. Last updated January 2017. London: NICE. Available from: https://www.nice.org.uk/guidance/cg70. [Accessed 14 April 2019].

Nursing and Midwifery Council (NMC), 2019. *Standards of proficiency for midwives*. London: NMC. Available from: https://www.nmc.org.uk/globalassets/sitedocuments/standards/standards-of-proficiency-for-midwives.pdf. [Accessed 20 November 2019].

Royal College of Obstetricians and Gynaecologists (RCOG), (2010). *GTG 55 Late intrauterine death and stillbirth* [online]. London, RCOG. Available from: https://www.rcog.org.uk/globalassets/documents/guidelines/gtg_55.pdf. [Accessed 23 June 2019].

Royal College of Obstetricians and Gynaecologists (RCOG), (2011). *Evidence-based Clinical Guideline 7 - The Care of Women Requesting Induced Abortion* [online]. London, RCOG. Available from: https://www.rcog.org.uk/globalassets/documents/guidelines/abortion-guideline_web_1.pdf. [Accessed 23 June 2019].

SmPC from the eMC. Cervagem® 1mg pessary. SANOFI. Last updated on the eMC 17/01/2014.

SmPC from the eMC. Cytotec® 200mcg tablets. Pfizer Ltd. Last updated on the eMC 26/07/2018.

SmPC from the eMC. Hemabate® sterile solution. Pfizer Ltd. Last updated on the eMC 10/10/2013.

SmPC from the eMC. Mifegyne® 200mg tablets. Exelgyn. Last updated on the eMC 11/08/2017.

SmPC from the eMC. Propess® 10mg vaginal delivery system. Ferring Pharmaceuticals Ltd. Last updated on the eMC 16/11/2017.

SmPC from the eMC. Prostin E$_2$® 1mg and 2mg Vaginal gel, and 3 mg Vaginal tablets. Pfizer Ltd. Last updated on the eMC 01/02/2018.

Tang, O., Gemzelle-Danielsson, K., & Ho, P. (2007). Misoprostol: pharmacokinetic profile, effects on the uterus and side-effects. *International Journal of Gynaecology and Obstetrics*, 99, S160–S167. Available from: http://www.misoprostol.org/downloads/misoprostol-journals/IJGO_pharm_Tang.pdf. [Accessed 18 June 2019].

Weiner, C., & Mason, C. (2017). Medication. In D. James, P. Steer, C. Weiner, B. Gonik, & S. Robson (Eds.), *High risk pregnancy: Management options* (5th ed.) (pp. 808–846). Cambridge: Cambridge University Press.

Rectal Preparations – Laxatives and Haemorrhoid Preparations

Laxatives

These are medicines that loosen the bowel content and encourage evacuation. They are also known as aperients. Use of certain laxatives in pregnancy and the puerperium is generally considered safe. When dietary and lifestyle changes or non-pharmacological preparations have failed or there are gastrointestinal or neurological conditions, there is a variety of pharmacological choices: bulk-forming agents, stimulant laxatives, stool softeners and osmotic preparations. Before prescribing laxatives it is important to ascertain that the patient is constipated and that the condition is not secondary to an underlying undiagnosed complaint.

Haemorrhoid Preparations

These come in the form of suppositories or topical creams and are made up of combinations of ingredients such as soothing compounds, e.g. local anaesthetic, and corticosteroids, e.g. hydrocortisone to alleviate the local inflammatory response; they may also contain mild astringents, vasoconstrictors and heparinoids to help relieve the haemorrhoid.

Anusol – cream, ointment, suppositories – applied twice daily after a bowel movement, or one suppository twice daily – use neither for longer than 7 days (eMC 13/4/2018)

Scheriproct – ointment or suppositories – apply twice daily for 5–7 days (3–4 times daily on first day if necessary), then once daily for a few days until symptoms have cleared, or one suppository daily after bowel movement for 5–7 days (eMC 3/4/2019)

Proctosedyl – ointment or suppositories – apply twice daily after bowel movement, or insert one suppository twice daily after bowel movement – do not use either for longer than 7 days (eMC 25/1/2019).

The student should be aware of:
- the effect of progesterone on the alimentary tract musculature
- factors predisposing to haemorrhoids
- the use of dietary and lifestyle measures to alleviate constipation and haemorrhoid discomfort
- regimes following surgical repair of third- or fourth-degree perineal trauma (see for example RCOG GTG 29, 2015).

BP
Bisacodyl

Proprietary
Dulcolax® (SANOFI)
Bisacodyl (non-proprietary, see BNF for details)

Group
Stimulant laxative

Uses/indications
Constipation

Type of drug
GSL

Presentation
Gastro-resistant tablets (GSL); smooth white torpedo-shaped suppositories (P)

Continued

Dosage

Tablet 5–10 mg nocte, action over 10–12 hours; one 10-mg suppository (eMC 3/1/2018)

Route of admin

Oral, P.R.

Contraindications

In patients with ileus, intestinal obstruction, acute abdominal conditions including appendicitis, acute inflammatory bowel diseases, and severe abdominal pain associated with nausea and vomiting, which may be indicative of the aforementioned severe conditions
In severe dehydration and in patients with known hypersensitivity to bisacodyl or any other component of the product
Should not be used when anal fissures or ulcerative proctitis with mucosal damage are present
Avoid use in children under 10 years
Should not be used for more than 5 consecutive days without investigating the cause of constipation

Side effects

Abdominal cramps; not for prolonged use as it can cause atonic non-functioning colon and hypokalaemia

Interactions

If used with antacids and milk products the resistance of the coating of the tablets may be reduced resulting in dyspepsia and gastric irritation

Pharmacodynamic properties

Stimulation of the mucosa of the large intestine results in colonic peristalsis with promotion of accumulation of water, and electrolytes, in the colonic lumen
This results in a stimulation of defaecation, reduction of transit time and softening of the stool
Stimulation of the rectum causes increased motility and a feeling of rectal fullness

Fetal risk
No data available but use only if the benefits out-weigh the risks

Breastfeeding
Considered safe but use only if the benefits outweigh the risks

BP
Docusate sodium

Proprietary
Norgalax® enema (Essential Pharma Ltd)
Docusate sodium (non-proprietary, see BNF for details)

Group
Stimulant laxative

Uses/indications
Constipation

Type of drug
P

Presentation
Rectal gel (enema)

Dosage
Active ingredient docusate sodium 0.12 g in each 10 g micro-enema; 1 micro-enema (120 mg/10 mg) if required (BNF 2019)

Route of admin
P.R.

Contraindications
Haemorrhoids, anal fissures, rectocolitis, anal bleed-ing, abdominal pain, intestinal obstruction, nausea, vomiting, inflammatory bowel disease, ileus and known hypersensitivity to any of the ingredients

Side effects
Anal burning, rectal pain, rectal bleeding, diarrhoea, urticaria, hepatotoxicity

Interactions
May increase the resorption of medicines
Not to be used in combination with hepatotoxic agents

Pharmacodynamic properties
Used as a faecal softening agent; considered to ease constipation by increasing the penetration of fluid into the faeces thereby causing them to soften
Norgalax® is usually effective in 5–20 min

Fetal risk
Use only if the benefits outweigh the risks

Breastfeeding
Use only if the benefits outweigh the risks

BP
Senna

Proprietary
Senokot® tablets or syrup (Forum Health Products Ltd)
Senna (as sennosides) (non-proprietary, see BNF for details)

Group
Stimulant laxative

Uses/indications
Constipation

Type of drug
P, GSL

Presentation
Tablets (brown)

Dosage
Tablets 7.5 mg as 7.5 mg to 30 mg nocte; syrup
7.5 mg/5 mL as 5-20 mL (eMC 23/9/2015)

Route of admin
Oral

Contraindications
Persistent abdominal symptoms
Avoid abuse as it can cause atonic non-functioning
colon and hypokalaemia

Side effects
Abdominal cramps, local irritation

Interactions
No data available

Pharmacodynamic properties
The sugar moiety of sennosides is removed by bacteria in
the large intestine, releasing the active anthrone fraction
This stimulates peristalsis via the submucosal and
myenteric nerve plexuses
Sennosides act in 8–12 hours

Fetal risk
No reports of fetal or animal toxicity

Breastfeeding
Standardized preparations are considered safe

BP
Glycerin

Proprietary
Glycerin suppositories (Thornton & Ross Ltd)
Glycerin suppositories (non-proprietary, see BNF for
details)

Group
Stimulant laxative – rectal stimulant only

Uses/indications
Constipation

Type of drug
GSL

Presentation
Suppositories

Dosage
Adult: 4 g = one suppository (eMC 13/1/2015)

Route of admin
P.R.; the suppository should be dipped in water before insertion

Contraindications
Anal fissure, haemorrhoids

Side effects
Local irritation

Interactions
None known

Pharmacodynamic properties
Promotes peristalsis and evacuation of the lower bowel by virtue of its irritant action

Fetal risk
Should be avoided in pregnancy unless directed by a physician

Breastfeeding
Should be avoided during lactation unless directed by a physician

---

BP
Lactulose solution

Proprietary
Duphalac® (Mylan Products Ltd)
Lactulose solution (non-proprietary, see BNF for details)

Group
Osmotic laxative

Uses/indications
Constipation

Type of drug
P

Presentation
A colourless to brownish yellow, clear or not more than slightly opalescent liquid

Dosage
Oral solution 3.335 g/5 mL as starting dose 15-45 mL with maintenance of 15 mL b.d. (eMC 7/11/2018)

Route of admin
Oral

Contraindications
Galactosaemia, intestinal obstruction

Side effects
Flatulence, abdominal cramps and discomfort

Interactions
No data available

Pharmacodynamic properties
The active ingredient, lactulose, is metabolized in the colon by the saccharolytic bacteria, producing low molecular weight organic acids, mainly lactic acid, that lower the pH of the colonic contents and promote the retention of water by an osmotic effect, thus increasing peristaltic activity

Fetal risk
No reports of teratogenicity or hazard to the fetus

Breastfeeding
Considered safe

Continued

BP
Liquid paraffin

Proprietary
Liquid Paraffin oral emulsion (non-proprietary, see BNF for details)

Group
Stool softener

Uses/indications
Temporary relief of constipation

Type of drug
P

Presentation
Liquid

Dosage
Adult: 10–30 mL when required (eMC 16/4/2015)

Route of admin
Oral

Contraindications
Children under 3 years of age

Side effects
Anal seepage of paraffin with consequent anal irritation after prolonged use
Granulomatous reaction caused by absorption of small quantities of liquid paraffin
Lipoid pneumonia (by accidental inhalation) may occur; therefore caution needed in patients with swallowing difficulty

Interactions
May interfere with the absorption of fat-soluble vitamins

Pharmacodynamic properties
Paraffin acts as a lubricant and penetrates and softens the stools

Fetal risk
Avoid during early pregnancy

Breastfeeding
Avoid during lactation

BP
Ispaghula husk

Proprietary
Fybogel® Orange or Lemon (Forum Health Products Ltd)
Ispaghula husk (non-proprietary, see BNF for details)

Group
Bulk-forming laxatives

Uses/indications
Those requiring a high-fibre regime, e.g. relief of constipation, including constipation in pregnancy and the maintenance of regularity, management of bowel function in patients with a colostomy, ileostomy, haemorrhoids, anal fissure, chronic diarrhoea associated with diverticular disease, irritable bowel syndrome and ulcerative colitis

Type of drug
GSL

Presentation
Effervescent granules

Dosage
A unit dose (one sachet or two level 5 mL spoonfuls) contains 3.5 g ispaghula husk; one sachet or two level 5 mL spoonfuls morning and evening (eMC 26/7/2017)

Route of admin
Oral

Continued

Contraindications

Intestinal obstruction, faecal impaction and colonic atony

Side effects

Minor abdominal distension and flatulence

Interactions

None known

Pharmacodynamic properties

Ispaghula husk is able to absorb up to 40 times its own weight in water in vitro, and part of its activity can be attributed to its action as a simple bulking agent
Additionally, colonic bacteria are believed to use the hydrated material as a metabolic substrate, resulting in an increase in the bacterial cell mass and resulting in softening of the faeces

Fetal risk

May be used during pregnancy as the ispaghula husk is not absorbed from the gastrointestinal tract

Breastfeeding

May be used during lactation as the ispaghula husk is not absorbed from the gastrointestinal tract

References and Recommended Reading

Briggs, G., Freeman, R., Towers, C., & Forinash, A. (2017). *Drugs in pregnancy and lactation: A reference guide to fetal and neonatal risk* (11th ed.). Philadelphia: Wolters Kluwer.

Dougherty, L., Lister, S., & West-Oram, A. (2015). *The Royal Marsden Manual of Clinical Nursing Procedures, Professional Edition, 9th ed. (Royal Marsden Manual Series)*. Chichester, West Sussex: Wiley Blackwell.

Johnson, R., & Taylor, W. (2016). *Skills for midwifery practice* (4th ed.). Edinburgh: Elsevier.

Jordan, S., & Hegarty, B. (2010). Laxatives in pregnancy and the puerperium. In S. Jordan (Ed.), *Pharmacology for midwives: The evidence base for safe practice* (2nd ed.) (pp. 272–283). Basingstoke: Palgrave Macmillan.

Norgalax 120mg/10g enema. Essential Pharma Ltd. Last updated on the BNF [online] April 2019.

Nursing and Midwifery Council (NMC), 2019. *Standards of proficiency for midwives*. London: NMC. https://www.nmc.org.uk/globalassets/sitedocuments/standards/standards-of-proficiency-for-midwives.pdf. [Accessed 20 November 2019].

Royal College of Obstetricians and Gynecologists (RCOG). (2015). *GTG 29 the management of third and fourth degree perineal tears [online]*. London: RCOG. https://www.rcog.org.uk/globalassets/documents/guidelines/gtg-29.pdf. [Accessed 4 July 2019].

SmPC from the eMC. Anusol® cream, HC ointment and HC suppositories. Church & Dweight UK Ltd. Last updated on the eMC 13/4/2018.

SmPC from the eMC. Dulcolax® 10 mg suppositories and 5 mg tablets. SANOFI. Last updated on the eMC 3/1/2019.

SmPC from the eMC. Duphalac® oral suspension. Mylan Products Ltd. Last updated on the eMC 7/11/2018.

SmPC from the eMC. Fybogel® Orange or Lemon granules (3.5 g ispaghula husk). Forum Health Products Ltd. Last updated on the eMC 26/7/2017.

SmPC from the eMC. Glycerin suppositories 4g (adult size). Thornton & Ross Ltd. Last updated on the eMC 13/1/2015.

SmPC from the eMC. Liquid Paraffin. Thornton & Ross Ltd. Last updated on the eMC 16/4/2015.

SmPC from the eMC. Proctosedyl® ointment and suppositories. SANOFI. Last updated on the eMC 25/1/2019.

SmPC from the eMC. Scheriproct® ointment and suppositories. Bayer PLC. Last updated on the eMC 3/4/2019.

SmPC from the eMC. Senokot® tablets and syrup. Forum Health Products Ltd. Last updated on the eMC 23/9/2015.

Thakar, R., & Sultan, A. (2017). Perineal repair and pelvic floor injury. In D. K. James, P. J. Steer, C. P. Weiner, B. Gonik, & S. Robson (Eds.), *High risk pregnancy: Management options* (5th ed.) (pp. 1843–1866). Cambridge: Cambridge University Press.

Weiner, C., & Mason, C. (2017). Medication. In D. K. James, P. J. Steer, C. P. Weiner, B. Gonik, & S. Robson (Eds.), *High risk pregnancy: Management options* (5th ed.) (pp. 808–846). Cambridge: Cambridge University Press.

24

Vaccines

A vaccine is a suspension of dead or disabled organisms that, when ingested or injected, prevents, lessens or treats infections or disease. The most commonly used vaccines in midwifery are rubella (the single antigen vaccine is no longer available in the UK), hepatitis B and Bacille Calmette–Guérin (BCG) vaccine. All women should be offered rubella screening in early antenatal care to identify the risk of contracting rubella infection; this enables MMR (measles, mumps, rubella) vaccination to be offered following birth and before discharge.

Serological screening for hepatitis B virus should be offered to pregnant women so that effective postnatal intervention can be offered to infected women to decrease the risk of mother-to-child transmission.

Vaccines are either live attenuated, which usually produce a durable immunity, although not necessarily as long-lasting as immunity resulting from natural infection, or inactivated; a series of injections of vaccine may be administered to produce an adequate antibody response.

The student should be aware of:

- detection of low levels of rubella antibodies in a client
- when it is appropriate to give vaccines in the postnatal period
- the sequelae of either vaccination or disease
- the possible side effects of vaccination.

BP
Rubella vaccine (as part of combined measles, mumps and rubella vaccine – MMR)

Proprietary
Priorix® (GlaxoSmithKline UK) (measles, mumps and rubella – MMR)

Group
Vaccine – live attenuated

Uses/indications
Vaccination where there are low levels of rubella antibodies or none detected

Type of drug
POM

Presentation
Ampoules, powder and solvent for reconstitution

Dosage
Dependent on age of recipient (eMC 24/1/2019)

Route of admin
S.C. or IM

Contraindications
Pregnancy or the intention to become pregnant within 1 month; febrile patients
Systemic hypersensitivity to any component of the vaccine or to neomycin
Extreme care if administered to individuals with egg allergy
Impaired immune function (however, recommend in asymptomatic HIV infection)

Side effects
A mild form of the disease
Rash or swelling at the injection site (use a lesion-free site if eczema)

Continued

Interactions

Possible interference from passive antibodies

Can be administered at the same time as the live varicella vaccine (Varilrix) but separate injection sites must be used

Priorix® cannot be given at the same time as other live attenuated vaccines; an interval of 4 weeks should be left between vaccinations

In individuals who have received human gamma globulins or a blood transfusion, vaccination should be delayed for at least 3 months owing to the possibility of vaccine failure due to passively acquired mumps, measles and rubella antibodies

If being given primarily to achieve protection against rubella, the vaccine may be given within 3 months of the administration of an immunoglobulin preparation or a blood transfusion

If tuberculin testing is required, it should be carried out before, or simultaneously, as it has been reported that live measles (and possibly mumps) vaccine may cause a temporary depression of tuberculin skin sensitivity resulting in inconclusive results

If alcohol swabs are used to cleanse the skin, the alcohol must be allowed to evaporate as it may inactivate the vaccine

Pharmacodynamic properties

Induces active immunization against rubella virus infection

Fetal risk

Theoretical risk of teratogenicity and should therefore be avoided unless the need for vaccination outweighs the risk to the fetus

Breastfeeding

Available data suggest that breastfeeding is safe

BP
Hepatitis B vaccine

Proprietary
Engerix B® (GlaxoSmithKline UK)
HBvaxPRO® (Merck Sharpe and Dohme Ltd)

Group
Vaccine

Uses/indications
Active immunization against hepatitis B virus infection (HBV) caused by all known subtypes in non-immune subjects

Type of drug
POM, Midwives' Exemptions

Presentation
Suspension for injection
Store between 2°C and 8°C

Dosage
Engerix B® 20 mcg/mL vial: IM adult and children over 16 years: 3 doses of 20 mcg, the second 1 month and the third 6 months after the first dose (eMC 24/4/2017)
HBvaxPRO® 10 mcg: Neonate (except if born to hepatitis B surface antigen (HBsAg)-positive mother, see below) and child 1 month to 16 years: 3 doses of 10 mcg, the second 1 month and the third 6 months after the first dose (eMC 12/3/2019)
Neonate born to HBsAg-positive mother (see note above): 4 doses of 10 mcg, first dose at birth with hepatitis B immunoglobulin (HBIg) injection (separate site) the second 1 month, the third 2 months and the fourth 12 months after the first dose (eMC 12/3/2019)
NB: see manufacturers' information and BNF for other schedules and information on boosters which may be recommended for immunocompromised patients

Continued

Route of admin
IM

Contraindications
Hypersensitivity

Side effects
Drowsiness, headache, nausea, vomiting, diarrhoea, abdominal pain, loss of appetite, pain and redness at injection site, fatigue, fever (≥37.5°C), malaise, swelling at injection site, injection site reaction (such as induration), influenza-like illness, irritability, apnoea in very premature infants (≤28 weeks' gestation)
NB: due to the risk of apnoea, respiratory monitoring for 48–72 hours should be considered when administering the primary immunization series to infants born at ≤28 weeks of gestation and particularly those with a previous history of respiratory immaturity
The benefit of vaccination is high in this group of infants, so vaccination should not be withheld or delayed

Interactions
Administration of Engerix B® and a standard dose of HBIg does not result in lower anti-HBs antibody titres provided they are administered at separate injection sites
Can be given together with *Haemophilus influenzae b*, BCG, hepatitis A, polio, combined measles, mumps and rubella as MMR, diphtheria, tetanus and pertussis vaccines

Pharmacodynamic properties
Induces specific humoral antibodies against HBsAg (anti-HBs antibodies)
An anti-HBs antibody titre ≥10 IU/L correlates with protection to HBV infection

Fetal risk
No evidence available; use only if benefits outweigh possible risks

Breastfeeding
No evidence to say unsafe

BP
Bacille Calmette–Guérin vaccine

Proprietary
BCG Vaccine (AJ Vaccines A/S)

Group
Live attenuated vaccine

Uses/indications
Active immunization against tuberculosis

Type of drug
POM

Presentation
Powder and solvent for suspension for reconstitution as injection

Dosage
Adults and children aged 12 months and over: 0.1 mL of the reconstituted vaccine; infants under 12 months of age: a dose of 0.05 mL of the reconstituted vaccine (eMC 11/10/2019)

Route of admin
Intradermal: if alcohol swabs are used to cleanse the skin, the alcohol must be allowed to evaporate as it may inactivate the vaccine

Contraindications
Hypersensitivity: postponed if pyrexia or generalized skin infection; those receiving systemic corticosteroids or immunosuppressive treatment; not to be given to patients who are receiving antituberculous drugs

Side effects

The expected reaction to successful vaccination with
BCG Vaccine includes induration at the injection site
followed by a local lesion that may ulcerate some
weeks later and heal over some months later, leaving
a small, flat scar

CAUTION: poor injection technique, overdose or an
excessive response may result in a discharging ulcer

Interactions

May be given concurrently with inactivated or live
vaccines, including combined measles, mumps and
rubella vaccines

If other vaccines are administered at the same time,
they should not be given into the same arm, or if not
given at the same time an interval of not less than 4
weeks is recommended

Advised not to give further vaccination into the same
arm used for BCG vaccination for 3 months due to
the risk of regional lymphadenitis

Pharmacodynamic properties

Causes a cell-mediated immune response that confers
a variable degree of protection to infection with
Mycobacterium tuberculosis

The duration of immunity after BCG vaccination is
not known, although it is considered that immunity
reduces after 10 years

Fetal risk

BCG may be given during pregnancy if the benefit
of vaccination outweighs the risk, or in populations
considered at high risk of tuberculosis

Breastfeeding

BCG may be given during lactation if the benefit
of vaccination outweighs the risk or in populations
considered at high risk of tuberculosis

References and Recommended Reading

Briggs, G., Freeman, R., Towers, C., & Forinash, A. (2017). *Drugs in pregnancy and lactation: A reference guide to fetal and neonatal risk* (11th ed.). Philadelphia: Wolters Kluwer.

Hepatitis, B., & Foundation, U. K. *Education About Hepatitis B for Health and Social Care Professionals*. Available from: http://www.hepb.org/assets/Uploads/Health-Care-Providers-Fact-Sheet2.pdf. [Accessed 16 April 2019].

Hepatitis, B., & Foundation, U. K. Factsheet for Hepatitis B and Pregnancy. Available from: http://www.hepb.org/assets/Uploads/Pregnancy-and-Hepatitis-B-Fact-Sheet-final.pdf. [Accessed 16 April 2019].

Jordan, S. (2010). *Pharmacology for midwives: The evidence base for safe practice* (2nd ed.). Basingstoke: Palgrave Macmillan.

Nuangchamnong, N., & Andrews, J. (2017). Hepatitis virus infections in pregnancy. In D. James, P. Steer, C. Weiner, B. Gonik, & S. Robson (Eds.), *High risk pregnancy: Management options* (5th ed.) (pp. 469–478). Cambridge: Cambridge University Press.

Nursing and Midwifery Council (NMC), 2019. *Standards of proficiency for midwives*. London: NMC. Available from https://www.nmc.org.uk/globalassets/sitedocuments/standards/standards-of-proficiency-for-midwives.pdf. [Accessed 20 November 2019].

Riley, L. (2017). Rubella, measles, mumps, varicella and parvovirus. In D. James, P. Steer, C. Weiner, B. Gonik, & S. Robson (Eds.), *High risk pregnancy: Management options* (5th ed.) (pp. 493–502). Cambridge: Cambridge University Press.

Roos, T., & Baker, D. (2017). Cytomegalovirus, herpes simplex virus, adenovirus, coxsackievirus and human papillomavirus. In D. James, P. Steer, C. Weiner, B. Gonik, & S. Robson (Eds.), *High risk pregnancy: Management options* (5th ed.) (pp. 503–520). Cambridge: Cambridge University Press.

Royal College of Obstetricians and Gynaecologists (RCOG). (2015). *GTG 13 Chickenpox in Pregnancy [online]*. London: RCOG. Available from: https://www.rcog.org.uk/globalassets/documents/guidelines/gtg13.pdf. [Accessed 16 April 2019].

SmPC from the eMC. BCG Vaccine AJV, powder and solvent for suspension for injection. AJ Vaccines A/S. Last updated on the eMC 11/10/2019.

SmPC from the eMC. HBVaxPRO® 10mcg in 1mL suspension in pre-filled syringe. Merck Sharpe and Dohme Ltd. Last updated on the eMC 12/3/2019.

SmPC from the eMC. Engerix B® 20 micrograms/1 ml vials for injection. GlaxoSmithKlein UK. Last updated on the eMC 24/4/2017.

SmPC from the eMC. Priorix® powder and solvent for injection in pre-filled syringe. GlaxoSmithKlein UK. Last updated on the eMC 24/1/2019.

Watts, D. (2017). Human immunodeficiency virus. In D. James, P. Steer, C. Weiner, B. Gonik, & S. Robson (Eds.), *High risk pregnancy: Management options* (5th ed.) (pp. 479–492). Cambridge: Cambridge University Press.

Weiner, C., & Mason, C. (2017). Medication. In D. James, P. Steer, C. Weiner, B. Gonik, & S. Robson (Eds.), *High risk pregnancy: Management options* (5th ed.) (pp. 808–846). Cambridge: Cambridge University Press.

Further Reading

Public Health England. Resources for Pregnancy Screening.

a) See   https://www.gov.uk/guidance/infectious-diseases-in-pregnancy-screening-programme-overview.

b) See antibiotic treatment (IM Penicillin) for syphilis infection

c) Link for leaflets https://www.gov.uk/government/collections/population-screening-programmes-leaflets-and-how-to-order-them

Vitamins and Iron Preparations

Vitamins

Vitamins are factors in food necessary for growth and reproduction of living tissues. Some vitamins are fat soluble and others are water soluble. Those of interest to the midwife are vitamins C, B_{12}, K and folic acid, and are usually present in a healthy and balanced diet.

Supplements of vitamins C and K are rare, but B_{12} and folic acid supplements remain popular generally but especially where restricted diets affect nutritional intake (NICE 2008a, NICE 2008b). More recently, vitamin D has been in the spotlight with the re-emergence of neonatal rickets and reduced mineralization within the bones of children within certain populations. National Institute for Health and Clinical Excellence (NICE) guidelines 2008c (updated 2019) add advice for specific populations.

Other elements present in food are minerals.

The student should be aware of:

- the importance of good nutrition in women of childbearing age
- what is considered malnutrition by the World Health Organization (WHO)
- the prevalence of malnutrition in local populations
- the appropriate provision of evidence-based information to improve the nutrition of women from a range of vulnerable groups, e.g. low income and disadvantaged families, women who have restrictive (medical, cultural or choice) diets

- the sequelae to mother and fetus of malnutrition
- the foods that are part of a well-balanced healthy diet
- current recommendations for supplementation for specific populations (see for example NICE 2006; NICE 2008a, NICE 2008b, NICE 2008c; NICE 2010).

Iron Preparations

Iron (Fe) is a metallic element and a constituent of the haemoglobin molecule that is necessary to carry oxygen around the body via the blood.

Vitamin C, and to a lesser extent folic acid, are involved in Fe absorption. In theory, the haemoglobin (Hb) concentration in the blood should increase by 2 g/100 mL, or 20 g/L, over 3–4 weeks of supplementation.

The student should be aware of:

- WHO guidelines for diagnosis of anaemia
- the aetiology of and predisposing factors for anaemia
- the physiology and pathophysiology of anaemia in pregnancy
- the appropriateness and effectiveness of Fe preparations, both in anaemia and routinely in pregnancy
- the different kinds of anaemia and their prognosis
- the dietary sources of Fe, vitamin B_{12}, vitamin C and folic acid
- the sequelae of anaemia in the antenatal, intranatal and postnatal periods.

NB: Because of the risk of anaphylactic reaction and cardiopulmonary collapse, Fe injections should be carried out under strict medical supervision. Resuscitation, defibrillation facilities and adrenaline (ephedrine) must be immediately available. It is also recommended that the course of oral Fe should be stopped 48 hours before the IM course.

A test dose is recommended prior to the first full administration.

Other Fe compounds

Pregaday® (RPH Pharmaceuticals AB) – ferrous fumarate (322 mg Fe) and folic acid (350 mcg) tablets (brown) – one tablet daily (BNF [online] 2019).

BP
Ferrous sulfate

Proprietary
Ferrous sulfate (Accord UK Limited)
Ferrous sulfate (non-proprietary, see BNF for details)

Group
Fe salts

Uses/indications
Iron deficiency anaemia

Type of drug
POM, GSL

Presentation
Tablets (white coated)

Dosage
One tablet = 200 mg dried ferrous sulfate equivalent to 65 mg elemental iron
One tablet 200 mg/day in prophylaxis or mild anaemia 2–3 tablets 130–195 mg/daily in divided therapeutic doses (BNF 2019)

Route of admin
Oral

Contraindications
Diverticulitis, inflammatory bowel disease, anaemias other than iron deficiency, concurrent administration of parenteral iron

Side effects
Nausea, gastric irritation, epigastric pain, diarrhoea or constipation, iron overload, darkening of the stools

---

Interactions

Antacids – magnesium trisilicate reduces the absorption of Fe

Antibiotics – absorption of antibiotics can be reduced in the presence of Fe

Methyldopa – possible reduction in the bioavailability of ferrous sulphate or ferrous gluconate if ingested with methyldopa

Pharmacodynamic properties

Iron aids haemoglobin regeneration and the oxidative processes in tissues

Fetal risk

No data available

Breastfeeding

Considered safe

BP

Iron dextran/sucrose compounds

Proprietary

CosmoFer® (Pharmacosmos UK Ltd)
Venofer® (Vifor Pharma UK Ltd)
Monofer® injection/infusion (Pharmacosmos UK Ltd)

Group

Fe salts

Uses/indications

Failure of oral therapy, i.e. severe continuous blood loss, malabsorption

Type of drug

POM

Presentation

Ampoules

Dosage

CosmoFer® – 50 mg/mL iron as ferrous hydroxide with dextran

Venofer® – 20 mg/mL iron as ferrous hydroxide with sucrose

Monofer® 100 mg/mL solution for injection/infusion – iron (III) isomaltoside 1000

Calculated according to client weight and iron deficiency – discontinue oral Fe 24 hours prior to injection

An example for CosmoFer® is 1.5 mg/kg body weight to a max 100 mg/day (eMC 23/1/2019)

Test dose of 25 mg to exclude anaphylactic reaction and remaining dose 60 min later (eMC 23/1/2019)

Route of admin

Deep IM (CosmoFer® only), slow IV or IV infusion: see manufacturers' recommendations for dilutants (IV and infusion)

Contraindications

Liver and kidney disease (pyelonephritis), untreated urinary tract infection, early pregnancy, pre-existing cardiac anomalies, existing asthma, allergic eczema or other atopic allergy should not be treated by IV injection; rheumatoid arthritis with active inflammation symptoms

Side effects

Anaphylactic reaction, pain at injection site, nausea, vomiting, dizziness, flushing, severe arrhythmias, theoretical risk of myocardial infarction, urine may turn black

Interactions

Chloramphenicol – may delay response to iron treatment; oral iron should not recommence until 5 days from last injection

Continued

Pharmacodynamic properties

Absorption from the injection site is rapid and complete, and therefore rapidly increases Fe stores for utilization as required

Fetal risk

May cause teratogenicity or abortion in early pregnancy; limit to second and third trimester recommended once risk/benefit assessed

Breastfeeding

No data, but manufacturers recommend avoidance

BP

Folic acid

Proprietary

Folic acid tablets (AAH Pharmaceuticals Ltd)
Folic acid (non-proprietary, see BNF for details)

Group

Vitamins – B complex

Uses/indications

Folate-deficient megaloblastic anaemia, pre-conception until 12 weeks' gestation, prevention of neural tube defects

Type of drug

POM, GSL (for GSL doses must not exceed 500 mcg/day)

Presentation

Tablets, syrup

Dosage

Pre-conception or first 12 weeks of gestation: 400 mcg daily (BNF 2019)
In folate-deficiency anaemia: 5 mg/day for 4 months or continued to term (BNF 2019)

Route of admin
Oral

Contraindications
Untreated pernicious anaemia or other cause of cobalamin deficiency, including lifelong vegetarians

Side effects
No data available

Interactions
Antiepileptics – absorption of phenytoin or phenobarbital is reduced (plasma concentrations), increasing the risk of seizures; therefore, advice should be taken on supplementation
Antibacterials – chloramphenicol and cotrimoxazole may interfere with folate metabolism

Fetal risk
No data available on overdosage

Breastfeeding
Actively excreted in breast milk; considered safe

BP
Vitamin B_{12} hydroxocobalamin acetate

Proprietary
Hydroxocobalamin (ADVANZ Pharma)
Hydroxocobalamin (non-proprietary, see BNF for details)

Group
Vitamins – B complex

Uses/indications
Very rare in pregnancy, pernicious anaemia, B_{12} deficiency

Continued

Type of drug
POM

Presentation
Glass ampoules

Dosage
1 mg, 3 times per week for 2 weeks; maintenance dose 1 mg every 3 months (eMC 17/1/2019)

Route of admin
Deep IM

Contraindications
Diagnosis of deficiency should be fully established

Side effects
Nausea, headaches, dizziness, fever, hypersensitivity and injection site reactions, hypokalaemia, and chromaturia

Interactions
Antiepileptics – reduced absorption of phenytoin or phenobarbital
Antibacterials – reduced response to chloramphenicol and cotrimoxazole

Fetal risk
Maternal B_{12} deficiency results in poor fetal outcome – there are no reports of high maternal dosage at *term* and maternal or fetal complications

Breastfeeding
Lack of B_{12} in the maternal diet can cause neonatal anaemia
Dietary supplements are recommended where deficiency is diagnosed

BP
Cholecalciferol (vitamin D_3)

Proprietary
Accrete D3 (Internis Pharmaceuticals Ltd), Adcal-D3
(Kyowa Kirin Ltd)

Group
Vitamins

Uses/indications
Calcium and vitamin D supplementation in at-risk
groups

Type of drug
POM

Presentation
Film-coated tablet/caplet – ochre/pale orange,
respectively

Dosage
400 IU/day (RCOG 2014a and RCOG 2014b guidance: In
general 400 units (or 10 mcg/day))
For high risk 1000 IU/day such as for women with
increased skin pigmentation, or have reduced exposure
to sunlight, or those who are socially excluded or obese
In cases of pre-eclampsia 800 IU/day is recommended
combined with calcium (see NICE 2014, RCOG
2014a).

Route of admin
Oral

Contraindications
Hypercalcaemia, hypercalciuria, renal disease, hypersensitivity to active substances, immobility

Side effects
Hypercalcaemia, hypercalciuria, abdominal pain, constipation, diarrhoea, nausea, flatulence, skin rashes

Continued

Interactions

Thiazide diuretics – reduced excretion of calcium

Tetracycline – calcium salts can interfere with tetracycline absorption

Cardiac glycosides – increased toxicity of cardiac glycosides, e.g. digitalis, oxalic acid (spinach, rhubarb and sorrel) and phytic acid (cereals) can reduce calcium absorption

Pharmacodynamic properties

Increases calcium absorption from intestine; counteracts parathyroid hormone production when calcium levels are depleted, cholecalciferol converted to 25-hydroxycholecalciferol in liver and 1,25-hydroxycholecalciferol in kidney, which increases calcium absorption

Fetal risk

Vitamin D: animal studies – toxicity at high doses

Calcium and vitamin D: prolonged hypercalcaemia may lead to impaired physical and mental development, supraventricular aortic stenosis and retinopathy

Breastfeeding

Calcium and vitamin D pass via breast milk, and this needs to be considered should supplements be required

References and Recommended Reading

Briggs, G., Freeman, R., Towers, C., & Forinash, A. (2017). *Drugs in pregnancy and lactation: A reference guide to fetal and neonatal risk* (11th ed.). Philadelphia: Wolters Kluwer.

Folic acid 400 mcg tablets. AAH Pharmaceuticals Ltd. Last updated on the BNF [online] April 2019.

Jordan, S. (2010). Nutritional supplements in pregnancy. In S. Jordan (Ed.), *Pharmacology for midwives: The evidence base for safe practice* (2nd ed.) (pp. 249–262). Basingstoke: Palgrave Macmillan.

National Institute of Health and Care Excellence (NICE). (2006). *CG37. Postnatal care up to 8 weeks after birth* [online]. Last updated 1 February 2015. London: NICE. Available from: https://www.nice.org.uk/guidance/cg37. [Accessed 14 April 2019].

National Institute of Health and Care Excellence (NICE). (2008a). *CG62 Antenatal care for uncomplicated pregnancies* [online]. Last updated February 2019. London: NICE. Available from: https://www.nice.org.uk/guidance/cg62. [Accessed 4 April 2019].

National Institute for Health and Clinical Excellence (NICE). (2008b). *PH11 Maternal and child nutrition* [online]. Last updated November 2014. London: NICE. Available from: http://www.nice.org.uk/guidance/ph11. [Accessed 19 April 2019].

National Institute for Health and Clinical Excellence (NICE). (2008c). *PH56 Vitamin D: Supplement use in specific population groups* [online]. Last updated August 2017. London: NICE. Available from: https://www.nice.org.uk/guidance/ph56. [Accessed 19 April 2019].

National Institute of Health and Care Excellence (NICE). (2010). *CG110. Pregnancy and complex social factors: A model for service provision for pregnant women with complex social factors* [online]. Last updated August 2018. London: NICE. Available from: https://www.nice.org.uk/guidance/cg110. [Accessed 14 April 2019].

National Institute of Health and Care Excellence (NICE). (2014). *PH56. Vitamin D: supplement use is specific population groups* [online]. Last updated August 2017 . Available from: https://www.nice.org.uk/guidance/ph56. [Accessed 4 April 2019].

Nursing and Midwifery Council (NMC), 2019. *Standards of proficiency for midwives*. London: NMC. Available from https://www.nmc.org.uk/globalassets/sitedocuments/standards/standards-of-proficiency-for-midwives.pdf. [Accessed 20 November 2019].

Royal College of Obstetricians (RCOG). (2014a). *Scientific Impact Paper 43 Vitamin D in Pregnancy* [online]. Available from: https://www.rcog.org.uk/globalassets/documents/guidelines/scientific-impact-papers/vitamin_d_sip43_june14.pdf . [Accessed 19 November 2019].

Royal College of Obstetricians (RCOG). (2014b). *GTG66 Management of Beta Thalassaemia in Pregnancy* [online]. Available from: https://www.rcog.org.uk/en/guidelines-research-services/guidelines/gtg66/. [Accessed 19 November 2019].

SmPC from the eMC. Accrete® D_3 tablets. Internis Pharmaceuticals Ltd. Last updated on the eMC 15/08/2016.

SmPC from the eMC. Adcal® D_3 chewable tablets. Kyowa Kirin Ltd. Last updated on the eMC 28/4/2017.

SmPC from the eMC. CosmoFer® solution for injection/infusion. Pharmacosmos UK Ltd. Last updated on the eMC 23/01/2019.

SmPC from the eMC. Ferrous Sulfate 200mg tablets. Accord-UK Ltd. Last updated on the eMC 25/07/2018.

SmPC from the eMC. Hydroxocobalamin® 1mg/mL solution for injection. ADVANZ Pharma. Last updated on the eMC 17/01/2019.

SmPC from the eMC. Monofer® 100mg/mL solution for injection/infusion. Pharmacosmos UK Ltd. Last updated on the eMC 09/06/2017.

SmPC from the eMC. Pregaday® 322mg/0.35mg film-coated tablets. RPH Pharmaceuticals AB. Last updated on the eMC 29/04/2019.

SmPC from the eMC. Venofer® solution for injection/infusion. Vifor Pharma UK Ltd. Last updated on the eMC 09/11/2016.

Soltani, H., & Fair, F. (2017). Nutrition and metabolism in pregnancy. In J. Rankin (Ed.), *2017. Physiology in childbearing with anatomy and related biosciences* (pp. 239–248). Edinburgh: Elsevier.

Weiner, C., & Mason, C. (2017). Medication. In D. James, P. Steer, C. Weiner, B. Gonik, & S. Robson (Eds.), *High risk pregnancy: Management options* (5th ed.) (pp. 808–846). Cambridge: Cambridge University Press.

World Health Organization. (2011). *WHO, Nutrition Experts Take Action on Malnutrition*. Available from: http://www.who.int/nutrition/pressnote_action_on_malnutrition/en/. [Accessed 16 April 2019].

World Health Organization. (2016). *WHO recommendations on antenatal care for a positive pregnancy experience*. Nutritional interventions, p14–39. Available from: https://www.who.int/nutrition/publications/guidelines/antenatalcare-pregnancy-positive-experience/en/. [Accessed 16 April 2019].

Further Reading

The Cochrane Library. Available http://www.thecochranelibrary.com/. [Accessed 16 April 2019] (various evidence-based information reviews on supplements in pregnancy and postnatal periods eg Keats, E., Haider, B., Tam, E. and Bhuttam Z., 2019. *Multiple-micronutrient supplementation for women during pregnancy.* Cochrane Systematic Review - Intervention).

26

Drug Calculations

The practitioner will need to be able to perform complex calculations in order that the correct volume or quantity of medications can be administered in all midwifery practice settings. It is good practice for a second (registered) professional to independently carry out the calculation to minimize the risk of error (RPS/RCN 2019, section 15, p. 4). Numerical skill and arithmetical knowledge are essential competencies for midwives, as the use of calculators should not substitute how volume and quantity are determined for safe standards of practice.

The student should be aware of:

- the NMC publications – *The Code* (NMC 2015), and *Practicing as a Midwife in the UK* (NMC 2017), and the RPS publications – *Professional Guidance for the Administration of Medicines in Healthcare Settings* (RPS/RCN 2019), and *Professional Guidance on the Safe and Secure Handling of Medicines* (RPS 2018).

- the NMC, (2019) publication Standards of proficiency for midwives and in particular the shared skills for evidence-based medicines administration and optimisation (principally Domains 3 and 4) (NMC 2019 p40).

- local NHS Trust guidelines for medicines management relating to administration

- drug calculation formulas used within their clinical practice (adult and neonatal) and competence in manipulation of numerical values within these formulas.

The Basic Formula

$$\frac{\text{required strength}}{\text{available strength}} \times \text{quantity preparation is supplied in}$$

or

$$\frac{\text{what you want}}{\text{what you've got}} \times \text{IT (the preparation)}$$

e.g. ampicillin elixir 125 mg/ mL – the prescription says 100 mg, therefore:

$$\frac{100}{125} \times 5 = 4 \text{ mL}$$

e.g. benzyl penicillin 600 mg/5 mL the prescription says 200 mg, therefore:

$$\frac{200}{600} \times 5 = 1.66 \text{ mL}$$

For Rates of Infusion

$$\text{Flow rate in mL/hr} = \frac{\text{Volume of fluid (mL)}}{\text{Time of infuse (hr)}}$$

e.g. Flow rate $= \dfrac{500}{8} = 62.5 = 63 \text{mL/h}$

If the infusion is to run over minutes then divide by the number of minutes to run:

$$\text{Flow rate in drops / min} = \frac{\text{mL to be infused}}{\text{hrs to be delivered}} \times \frac{\text{no. of drops per mL}}{\text{time in minutes (60)}}$$

e.g. 1 L fluid over 12 h, using a burette (60 drops/mL):

$$\text{Flow rate} = \frac{1000}{12} \times \frac{60}{60} = 83 \text{ drops/min}$$

e.g. 450 mL blood over 3 h using a blood-giving set (15 drops/mL):

$$\text{Flow rate} = \frac{450}{3} \times \frac{15}{60} = 37.5 = 38 \text{ drops/min}$$

An alternative mode of calculation that may be used utilizes a drop rate denominator (DRD):

$$\text{DRD} = \frac{\text{No. of drops per mL delivered by administration set (drop factor)}}{\text{No. of minutes in 1 h (i.e. 60 min)}}$$

60 drops per mL = 1 DRD

20 drops per mL = 3 DRD

15 drops per mL = 4 DRD

12 drops per mL = 5 DRD

10 drops per mL = 6 DRD

e.g. 450 mL blood over 3 h using a blood-giving set (15 drops/mL):

$$\text{Flow rate} = \frac{450}{3} = 150$$

$$\text{Then , } 150/(\text{DRD}) = \frac{150}{4} = 37.5 = 38 \text{ drops per min}$$

Neonatal Calculation

Students should also be able to use a formula that requires doses to be calculated from measures of weight.

e.g. neonatal paracetamol suspension – dose 10 mg/kg. So, for an infant weighing 3 kg (or 3000 g), the dose required would be 30 mg. Paracetamol suspension is 120 mg in 5 mL:

$$\frac{\text{what you want}}{\text{what you've got}} \times \text{IT (the preparation)}$$

$$\text{i.e. } \frac{30 \text{ mg}}{120 \text{ mg}} \times 5 \text{ mL} = 1.25 \text{ mL}$$

References and Recommended Reading

Lapham, R., & Agar, H. (2015). *Drug calculations for nurses – a step-by-step approach* (4th ed.). Boca Raton, Florida: CRC Press and Taylor Francis Group.

Nursing and Midwifery Council (NMC). (2015). *The code - professional standards of practice and behaviour for nurses, midwives and nursing associates*. Last updated 2018. London: NMC.

Nursing and Midwifery Council (NMC). (2017). *Practicing as a midwife in the UK*. Last updated 2019. London, NMC.

Nursing and Midwifery Council (NMC). (2019). *Standards of proficiency for midwives*. London: NMC. Available from: https://www.nmc.org.uk/globalassets/sitedocuments/standards/standards-of-proficiency-for-midwives.pdf. [Accessed 20 November 2019].

Royal Pharmaceutical Society and Royal College of Nursing (RPS/RCN). (2019). *Professional guidance for the administration of medicines in healthcare settings*. London, RPS: Endorsed by RCM.

Royal Pharmaceutical Society (RPS), Royal (2018). *Professional guidance on the safe and secure handling of medicines*. Available from: https://www.rpharms.com/recognition/setting-professional-standards/safe-and-secure-handling-of-medicines/professional-guidance-on-the-safe-and-secure-handling-of-medicines. [Accessed 12 April 2019].

Wright, K. (2011). *Drug calculations for nurses: Context for practice*. Basingstoke: Palgrave McMillan.

Wright, K., & Shepherd, E. (2017). How to calculate drug doses and infusion rates accurately. *Nursing Times [online]*, 113(10), 31–34. Available from: https://www.nursingtimes.net/clinical-archive/medicine-management/how-to-calculate-drug-doses-and-infusion-rates-accurately/7021671.article. [Accessed 19 April 2019].

Further Reading

clinicalskills.net Available from: www.clinicalskills.net/. [Accessed 19 April 2019].

Baston, H., Renton, M., Henshaw, A.-M., Hall, J., & Henley-Einion, A. (2009). *Midwifery essentials: Basics* (Vol. 1). Edinburgh: Churchill Livingstone.

Dougherty, L., Lister, S., & West-Oram, A. eds. (2015). *The Royal Marsden Manual of Clinical Nursing Procedures, Professional Edition, 9th ed. (Royal Marsden Manual Series)*. Chichester, WSussex, Wiley Blackwell.

Johnson, R., & Taylor, W. (2016). *Skills for midwifery practice* (4th ed.). Edinburgh: Elsevier.

INDEX

Note: Page numbers followed by "b" indicate boxes.